"As an author and international speaker, I meet many amazing coaches, trainers, authors and inspirational leaders. When I met Karen McCoy, I instantly realized this woman was in a league of her own. Her passion for health and fitness is driven not by vanity or ego -- although she looks very much like a world-class athlete. Karen is a living example of channelling her struggles and feelings of fear and loss into a life-enhancing, productive, empowered, healthy way of living, loving, moving, giving and receiving. Her book, **One Rep at a Time**, *pulls together everything one would need to feel physically, emotionally and spiritually strong!"*

— Crystal Andrus, bestselling author, founder of The SWAT Institute

*"***One Rep at a Time** *is an explicit and inspirational account of one woman's challenge to overcome the unexpected. Karen McCoy displays amazing courage and adaptability in her personal journey of self-discovery. Her life story proves that mental and physical health are both dependent on the resolution of much deeper emotional and spiritual concerns.* **One Rep at a Time** *draws the reader in with the power of authenticity and then provides a multi-dimensional solution for life based on health, nutrition and fitness science. This book teaches how to obtain a state of robust tranquility and inner peace through the acceptance of life as it is, not as it should or could be. It will strike your soul and touch you where it matters most."*

— Dr. Cory Holly, president, Cory Holly Institute

One Rep at a Time

An athlete and mother reveals the secrets
to creating inner power and serenity

KAREN McCOY

Introducing the
8-Week BLISS™ Body Makeover Program
to get you lean, fit, shapely and sexy for life!

For rights information and bulk orders, please contact
info@agiopublishing.com *or go to* www.agiopublishing.com

One Rep at a Time
ISBN 978-1-897435-70-0 (trade paperback)
ISBN 978-1-897435-71-7 (ebook)
Cataloguing information available from
Library and Archives Canada.
Printed on acid-free paper.
Agio Publishing House is a socially responsible company,
measuring success on a triple-bottom-line basis.
10 9 8 7 6 5 4 3 2 1

PUBLISHING HOUSE
151 Howe Street, Victoria BC Canada V8V 4K5

For Tristan,

who has taught me that true strength
is not measured by one's muscle.
It is measured by one's heart.
Wherever you go, I will always be there.

ACKNOWLEDGEMENTS

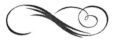

First, I wish to thank Truman Hoszouski who encouraged me to lift my first weight, over thirty years ago. You helped me bust through the stereotypes surrounding women and weights, and you helped me find my true calling. Your sheer passion for lifting has stayed with me all these years. Thank you, wherever you are.

To my husband, Neil, who has walked with me through many a dark night. Your patience and love, and your ability to see the good in me even when I couldn't, has kept me going. You are my rock, my safe place. I love you.

To my sister Sheryl, who has always been there for us. Thank you for all your support. You will always be Tristan's favourite Auntie.

To my father, Sherwood, who has long left this physical world. You instilled in me a love of music, a love of writing, and the importance of never, ever giving up. I only wish I'd had more time with you. I miss you.

To Bruce Batchelor, who painstakingly went over my manuscript and helped carve it into something I could truly be proud of. You've helped make me a better writer, and I thank you.

A special thank you to Cory and Tracy Holly. You truly walk the walk, and your commitment to living your truth is an inspiration to all. Thank you for all you've taught me.

To Crystal Andrus, who encouraged me to tell the real story, my story. You are a walking, breathing example of living life to the fullest and encouraging other women to do the same. You are a true angel.

To Tracey Harper of Fusion Artistry. Your beautiful photographs helped bring our story to life in a profound way. You are truly a gifted visionary.

To Marsha Batchelor who made the book a piece of art. Thank you for your guidance.

To Dan Batchelor who created the book's exercise videos. You have a very long and promising career ahead of you. Keep it up! I can't wait to see where your path leads you.

Many thanks to The Body Barn Gym, for letting us film there. Hopefully we didn't disrupt things too much!

To Muscular Dystrophy Canada for your continued support of all families living with neuromuscular disease.

To The Victoria Foundation for your long-standing dedication to philanthropy, and your support in helping our family create The Tristan Graham Children's Foundation.

A long overdue thank you to Jane Goranson-Coleman and Cheryl Forrest for introducing me to the power of the unseen world. Your teachings have been instrumental to my healing and growth, and they have paved the way for all that I do. May the Universe continue to work through you in mysterious ways.

To my spiritual 'team' of advisors. I don't see you, but I always feel your presence. Thank you for being patient with me, even when I didn't believe. I'm finally listening.

To all the women I've had the pleasure of training over the years, my deepest gratitude. You are *my* inspiration, and your commitment to something greater is truly inspiring. Keep lifting and keep loving with equal force.

A special heart-felt thank you to all the mothers who struggle with children with illness. It's a lonely, tiring road, to be sure, but know that there is so much more beyond what you can see. Reach out for help, and be gentle with yourself. You *are* enough.

Finally, to my son Tristan. I have loved you before you were born and I'll love you until the end of time. You have truly saved me. You are my reason for being here. Thank you for letting me share this amazing journey with you. I am truly honoured.

TABLE OF CONTENTS

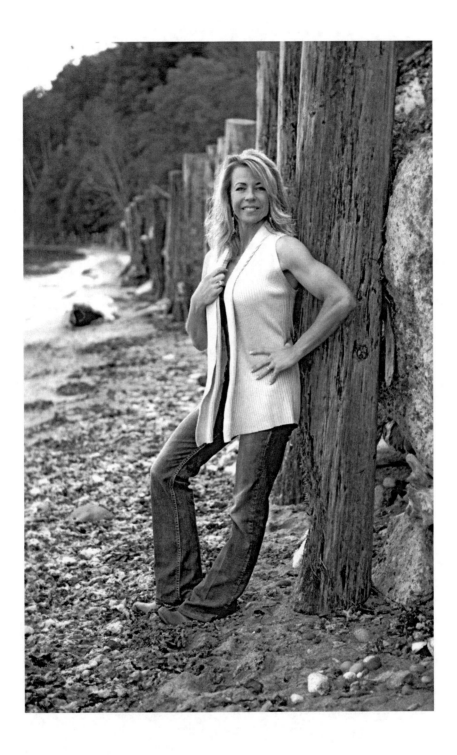

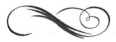

I Love Muscle

I love watching it move. For me, muscle represents life and vitality. It's graceful and sensual. It oozes health and confidence.

As a competitive bodybuilder, it was only natural that I write a fitness book. In fact, this book was originally written as a how-to training book about a year ago. Then I threw it out and started again. I needed to tell the real story, my story, of what real health and wellness means to me and to women everywhere.

One Rep at a Time is a book about women and health told from a very different place. It is carved out from that most mysterious of all journeys, the *dark night of the soul* – as described by mystic John of the Cross – that moment in time when we are faced with seemingly insurmountable challenges that offers us a kind of rebirth, and the chance to live life from a greater place. It's a journey we must all take toward wholeness, perhaps more than once, in order for us to live our best life physically, mentally, emotionally and spiritually.

I have spent most of my life teaching women how to build strong, shapely muscle, yet I gave birth to a child with a terminal muscle-wasting disease. The irony has not been lost on me. Looking back, I see that I had no choice really. This story needed to be told and I had to tell it for women everywhere.

My own dark night spanned eight years when my son was first diagnosed. Needless to say, I was ill-equipped for the ride. My body, which had once been my pillar of strength, became the focal point for all my anger, fear and confusion, and I lived in constant pain. I had to learn how to listen to its language, and open up to my journey in order to heal. Our bodies hold all our past stories, and I was a walking, breathing example of this, and so are you.

In today's exercise-crazed world, most of us have missed the point: building great abs is great, certainly, but it's not going to fix a broken marriage, or change destructive habits, or help us understand the connection between emotional pain and physical pain. We are multi-dimensional beings whose intuitions, dreams and energies are powerful tools we can use to create a strong, vibrant body and spirit, and build a life of meaning and purpose. I say we best get on with the journey.

That's why I've included in this book the **8-Week BLISS™ Body Makeover Program**, complete with videos and workout cards, and nutrition and lifestyle teachings to help you every step of the way. This is my thirty years of healthy living all wrapped up lovingly into one program, with hard-won lessons from my own life, which I know many of you will relate to. I guarantee you it is unlike any other exercise program you will ever encounter.

For me, my sport of choice has always been weight training, because I believe in that above all other exercise regimes. The skills required to build a strong, shapely body are the same skills needed to overcome intense challenges – strength, tenacity, focus, dedication and faith. The simple act of grabbing a weight and lifting it up is life-affirming. It's simple, clean and succinct. There's a start and an end. It doesn't get any more basic than that.

Life is hard. Few of us get through life unscathed, but surviving your own dark night means opening up to what is. It's about the intimate dance between holding on and letting go, and embracing its lessons. You learn to live fearlessly and with an open heart, and you learn to muscle into every moment like it was your last, because it just may be. This my son's journey has taught me.

Life isn't always lived in giant leaps and bounds. It's often lived in the small steps in between, the good and the bad ones, the glad and the sad ones, and the ones we often take for granted.

Sometimes life is lived just one step at a time … and *One Rep at a Time*.

With much love and respect,

PART I

THE JOURNEY

ONE

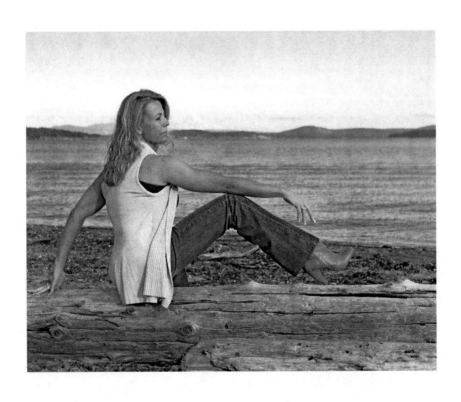

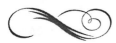

Women and Power:
First Lessons (1961 – 1981)

THE DIAGNOSIS, MAY 25, 2001

A big piece of me died today. A week ago, my son went for blood work. We had known for some time that he wasn't as strong as the other kids – stairs were tough for him and he ran with an awkward gait – but when the specialist ordered blood tests, I knew it was serious. A firm diagnosis could not be made for about three months, but the specialist suspected something, and he wouldn't tell me what.

Tristan had elevated levels of something called 'CPK' in his blood. I went home and looked it up. Elevated CPK is found in children with Duchenne Muscular Dystrophy (DMD), a fast-progressive and terminal muscle-wasting disease. My world began to unravel.

I called the doctor and demanded he tell me all what he suspected.

"Duchenne muscular dystrophy," he confirmed, "but thank goodness we caught it early enough."

I didn't understand. It wouldn't make any difference. There were no cures for DMD.

The doctor then began to tell me (over the phone) what would happen over the next 10 years: Tristan's muscles would continue to break down and he would be in a wheelchair by 9 or 10 years of age. He eventually wouldn't be able to bathe, feed or dress himself, and his heart and lungs would weaken. He would be on a respirator by his late teens, and our son would likely be gone in his twenties.

My head was spinning and I couldn't catch my breath. I asked him to slow down, please. I screamed and grabbed tightly onto the door jam. My partner ran into the room and caught me before I fell.

"I know this is a lot to take in," the doctor said, "but you have to know all this."

I screamed into the phone.

The following week we met at the doctor's office for the final confirmation. Tristan's father sat on one side of me, and my partner on the other.

"I'm sorry but the tests came back positive," the doctor said. "Your son has DMD."

We sat in silence.

Then the doctor turned to me and said, "I'm sorry, Mom."

I stared out the window and nodded. I wondered why the sun was still shining.

We walked out of the office and my partner went to get the truck. My ex and I sat in the lobby. He turned to me with tears in his eyes and said, "Promise me one thing, that you'll honour traditional things with our son, build memories, like Christmas stockings and Easter bunnies. I want him to know that when he leaves us, and he will leave us, that he was loved." He dropped his head and cried.

I promised I would.

For weeks I read everything I could about the disease. At night, when my son fell asleep, I would sneak into his room, lie down beside him and caress his tiny chest. I prayed to God that He give me the disease and spare my son. All I heard was silence.

Sleep did not come easy, if at all, so night after night I walked the streets in the pouring rain. It was like the sky was crying. I walked through the playground where Tristan often played, and I would sit among the cheery red, blue and yellow climbing pieces, and cry for the little boy for whom the struggle would only get more difficult, until one day he would no longer be able to climb – or walk – at all.

Beyond the playground was a path through an overhang of larch trees. I would stop and look up to the sky and say, "Walk with me, God." And we walked, He and I, and I would demand to know why this was happening. "Why Tristan? Why us?" I would ask. But there were no answers, only the sound of the rain falling.

When I'm asked to describe how I felt when I first heard the news, it was like an avalanche letting go: when the snow pack first breaks, you hear a loud Crack! then there's that 3-second delay before the snow pack releases and starts its slide down the mountainside. It was like that for me. I heard the doctor's words, I felt the Crack! in my body, then a few seconds later, I felt a heaviness slide into every muscle in my body. And there it would sit – like cement – for eight painful years.

My darkest night had begun. The journey was hard, and the lessons did not come easy. This is my story.

NATURE'S CHILD

I was brought up near Toronto, Ontario. My mother was a homemaker and my dad was a successful entrepreneur. My backyard consisted of acres of woods situated directly below the Niagara Escarpment with bits of the trail meandering through our property. Those woods were my playground, and I spent many hours playing in wood piles, building forts, and making tree swings within my natural environment.

I loved the freedom of the outdoors, and all its creatures that lived there. Hardly a summer would go by when I wouldn't find some small critter to mother – a chipmunk with a hurt back, a mole caught in the stream's current, baby mice abandoned by their mother or a bird who flew into a window and who now lay stunned on the ground.

Weekends we went to our cottage, and I spent most of my time in the water; we spent hours cruising the different lakes and shores in my dad's motorboat. For me, being anywhere near water was pure heaven. It was where I felt the most peaceful and grounded.

My fondest memories were the many gatherings at our home that were always built around good food and great music. My dad came from a long line of musicians, and his passion for music, mostly jazz music, was evident. There was always music playing in the background, and whenever we had guests for dinner, they were always trying to be heard over the music.

His love of music was passed on to me and at seven years old, I started playing the piano, like my grandparents and their parents before them. Music touched my sensitive nature, and when I played, I felt a kind of connection to everything. I loved the dedication and focus required to bring a sheet of music to life. Closing my eyes, I can still smell that old piano and feel its cool ivory keys under my fingertips.

FAMILY SECRETS (1972)

When I was 11 years old, my world changed forever. I was sitting in the family room when my mother got the call. She started to scream and shake. She slammed down the phone and turned to me and said, "Your father and I are getting a divorce."

Later, we learned that my father had confessed to my mother that he had another wife and child across town whom he had been living with for the past six years! Why my father wanted to come clean after so many years, I'll never know, but to make matters worse he now wanted his children to meet their new step-mother and half-brother. So we three kids piled into his car and arrived at his 'other' home.

As I walked through their house, I felt like I was in a movie. Everyone was so calm, and I remember thinking, *am I the only one who thinks this is absurd*? When I reached my new half-brother's bedroom, I leaned into the door and I stood in shock: there, on his bedroom shelves, were all the same toys and gifts my father had given me over the years. *I'm not special*, I thought. I felt all my power drain from my body. The betrayal cut my heart like a knife. Forty years later, I can still feel its sting.

My simple life as I knew it was over. My sister and brother and I packed up and moved to the city with our mom, while Dad and his other wife and son moved into our old home. It was hard leaving the home I loved, and even harder leaving my school. I simply wasn't ready to leave.

MY DE-THRONING

From the moment I arrived in my new school, it was a disaster. Being a sensitive and shy country girl didn't help and I just didn't feel like I belonged with these city kids. Just a few months previously, I was a popular and well-liked student at my old school – now I felt extremely awkward and out of sync. It was a lonely and confusing time for me.

Several months later, my mother announced that my sister, my brother and I would be moving *back* to our old house with my dad, step-mom and half-brother now living there, and we would be returning to our old school. I was confused but also excited to be going back to what I knew.

My first day back at my old school was the worst day of my young life. In my absence, my old friends had turned on me, and they threw me dirty looks when I walked past them in the hallway. I could hear them talking about my dad's 'other' family, and they snickered at me as I went by. Our family had become the talk of the town, and I was paying for it.

MY CINDERELLA LIFE (1974)

I was now 13 years old and although I'd always been an A-student, I found myself struggling with school. I hid in my room listening to music and writing poetry. And I ate. My favourite snack food was rice crispy squares, and I would make trays of squares and snack on them all night long. I hid my growing body under big, baggy shirts. My body had become my dumping ground for all my anger and depression, and the sadder I became, the bigger I got.

My mother moved far away and she remarried, and we only saw her twice a month. Her new husband had fallen on hard times, and after his divorce he began to drink heavily. His late-night alcoholic tirades were escalating. He had become physically abusive with my mother, and he had started to hurl his verbal assaults at me. I desperately wanted my mother to leave him, and for us all to return to our old way of life.

Back home, I resented being told what to do by my new step-mother and had become defiant. Her temper was fierce, and in an effort to protect myself, I had learned to fight back. Our yelling matches were of epic proportions, and our house trembled with the sounds of slamming doors. Sometimes things would escalate into physical brawls, which would leave us all feeling bruised for weeks afterward.

I was feeling engulfed by it all and, in an attempt to hold fast to whatever parts of myself I could, I became stubborn. But the more stubborn I became, the more discipline I got. I was not allowed to go out at night, or to have a job or spend money, and I wasn't allowed any friends over. My parents often grounded me for weeks on end, and I spent many weekends alone in my room. They started to criticize my weight and how I dressed, and I retreated further into myself. I felt powerless. I fell into a depression that lasted my teenage years.

I started smoking and hanging out with the wrong crowd, and we would often skip school to hang out at the mall. School, once a place where I excelled, now was just another way for my parents to try to control my life. So I rebelled against it and all that it represented.

The school principal called my parents to tell them that I was at risk of failing due to so many absences. My parents dug in their heels and dished out even harder discipline. I was to clean our house twice a week, wash all the family dishes after every meal (even if I didn't eat), and serve my parents coffee and snacks in their bedroom. My brothers were too young to know any different, and my sister had finally had enough and she left home before high school finished. I had become my parents' Cinderella.

FREEDOM (1979)

At 18 years old, I hated my life. It was January and I was graduating from high school at the end of the month, and I desperately wanted to leave home, but I didn't have a job or money. A girlfriend was flying to Banff, Alberta, for a ski holiday and I told my parents that once I finished school, I was going with her. They told me I couldn't, but I explained to them that I was now 18, and my grandmother had given me some money for a plane ticket. My dad was furious with me.

Three days later, my friend and I flew to Alberta. My father didn't talk to me for a full year.

When we arrived in Banff, I felt like I was truly *home*. I fell in love with the mountains, and for the first time in years, I felt free, with no one to criticize or control me. I had found my paradise. After ski season was over, my girlfriend returned home, and I stayed behind. I was living my life on my terms, and I vowed never to return home again.

I worked for a brief time as an elevator girl at the Banff Springs Hotel, then I applied at a popular pub downtown and I was immediately hired on. I loved my new life and I was enjoying my independence and making my own money. The staff was like one big family, and we spent most of our time together. I was 18 years old, and I was happy again.

THE MIRROR AT THE END OF THE HALL

One morning I went to pick up a co-worker at her apartment. As I walked toward her door, I caught my reflection in the full-length mirror at the end of the hall. I stopped and stared at myself. I was wearing purple terrycloth shorts and a yellow tank top, and I didn't like what I saw. My legs looked like carrot sticks, wide at the top and skinny at the ankle, with no shape or tone to them.

I'm not sure why I was so bothered by my reflection that morning, but it changed my life forever. Perhaps it was because I was living in one of the fittest cities in Canada, among world class athletes. I had come to appreciate the active lifestyle, but more importantly, I came to appreciate an athlete's dedication and hard work – and I loved how they looked. I marveled at the powerful thighs of a cyclist, the hard forearms of a rock climber, and the tight glutes of a downhill skier. Looking at my reflection, I saw none of that.

I had started running, biking and swimming, but my body's shape hadn't changed much. I wanted what those athletes had: the shape and tone, and the fact that they were doing something they loved. I wanted to be able to find something where I could channel all my energy and passion. I wanted to feel powerful and strong, like those athletes, and I wanted to look like them *too*.

IN THE GARAGE

The following year, I fell for an older guy who loved Harley David-son motorcycles and body building. He had a make-shift gym in his garage and he had welded together his own equipment. There were overhead cables, a leg press, a bench press and a preacher curl, and several sets of dumbbells and barbells.

One day as I was watching him train, I leafed through the latest issue of *Muscle & Fitness* magazine and I saw a picture of a woman lifting weights. I was amazed at her strong, tight arms and her shape-ly shoulders. Her name was Susie Green, and she was a model who used weight training to stay in shape.

I was in awe. I wanted what she had. I wanted her shape, her lines, and her confidence! My boyfriend could see the sparkle in my eye, and he insisted that I could easily look like her if I lifted weights. In those days, women training with weights were not the norm, but that made it all the more attractive to me! I couldn't wait to get started!

In that era, all the training programs in the magazines catered to men.

"Just train like them," my boyfriend said.

I said I didn't want to look like a man.

"Don't worry," he laughed. "You won't. You're a woman, you're not a man. You'll be more feminine than you ever imagined. Just lift as heavy as you can."

A RETURN TO POWER

From the moment I lifted my first weight, I was hooked. The feeling of control and connection was intoxicating and I loved every moment of it. I loved feeling the rush of blood into the muscles, and feeling my skin tighten as my muscles became engorged. I loved the metallic smell of the plates and the feel of the serrated metal collars of the dumbbells in my hands as I lifted them up over, and over again. I felt strong and powerful and in control of my body – and my life – again. I was unstoppable!

Day after day, I followed the men's training programs and I wrote everything down in a journal. I learned about the body builder's diet (which is what we call *clean eating* today) and the importance of proper hydration. I became an avid reader of all things related to weight training. In my mind's eye, I had a clear inner vision of my new body, with all its new curves, and I envisioned one day competing on stage.

FOREARMS

I remember the first time I noticed a new muscle on my body. I was reaching up for a bottle on a shelf and the light reflected off my forearm. There was a new thickness to my forearm muscles, and I stood there, clenching and unclenching my fist as I watched the tiny extensors in my forearm tighten and release. It was the smallest of movements, but my hard work was paying off! My body was starting to change!

For the next few weeks, I tore pictures out of body building magazines and thumb-tacked them up on the garage wall. Most of the pictures were men, but there were a handful of women entering the sport – Rachel McLish, Carla Dunlop, Laura Creavalle, Tonya Knight and Cory Everson – and I placed their pictures up alongside the men's. They were my inspiration to a new body and a new life.

CARDIO QUEENS

In the early '80s, cardio still ruled the day. Most women were into aerobics or running, but I was no longer interested in either. Although I had done both for several years, and my body had gotten smaller and I had dropped a lot of my teenage weight, my body hadn't *changed* much.

I wanted to really carve and shape my body in new ways. I had seen what weight training could do for a woman's body, and I just *knew* that was what I wanted. So day after day, I trained in our tiny, home-made gym, and was beginning to see a noticeable difference in my arms, in particular my biceps, which had become full and tight. Other areas were slower to show – in particular my butt and stomach, because this was where I had always carried my weight – but I wasn't about to give up.

GOING HOME

It had been two years since I left home, and I decided it was time to go back for a visit. My dad and step-mom were still unhappy with me because I decided to stay out west, so our visit was uncomfortable. They also learned that I was no longer playing piano which my father was very upset about. I loved my piano playing, but it had come to represent my parent's last hold-out over me. I needed to let the piano go in order to finally be free, and so I quit playing. It was my final act of defiance.

I didn't want to tell my family I started weight training, so I snuck off to the gym to train. One day, a male trainer came up to me and told me to leave.

I asked him why, and he said I was "... *a diversion to the male clientele.*"

With gym bag in had, I quickly left the gym. I felt humiliated and embarrassed. I couldn't wait to get back out west and to the safety of my home gym.

THROUGH THE LOOKING GLASS

As I continued to live and train in my beautiful mountain resort, I slowly cut the ties with my parents. I wanted to forget my childhood, and in my rush to move on with my life, I was just stuffing my childhood pain deeper inside of me. But all pain needs to be expressed in order to be released, and my body was to be the venue.

My past was about to re-surface in ways that I was clearly not prepared for.

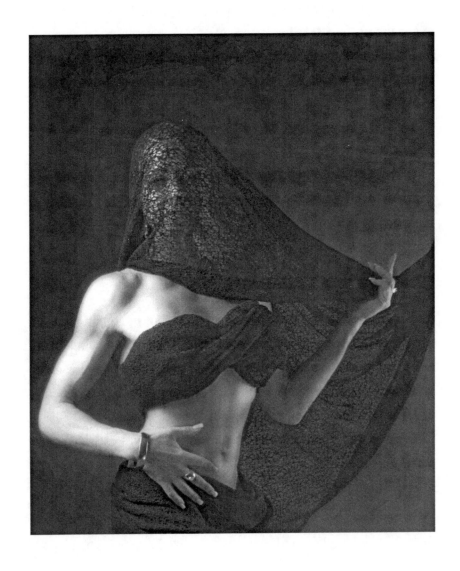

TWO

Behind the Veil:
New Glasses (1981 – 1999)

THE MOSQUITO CATCHER, JULY 7, 2001
(two months after diagnosis)

My son long ago made a rule in our household that we do not kill bugs. Instead, we gather up pesky flies and mosquitoes in a glass jar and release them outside. It's an agreement that includes ants, spiders, mosquitoes and all creepy crawlies.

Today I dropped Tristan off for his first day of summer camp. There was a swirl of worried parents, fretting camp leaders, and crying children not wanting to leave their parents' sides. Tristan seemed undisturbed by all the fuss. He quietly walked over to a pile of coloured Lego™ pieces and began to piece them together. He seemed to be a calming force that other kids gravitated towards, and soon he had a group of kids joining in. He asked me how long before I had to go and I said 10 minutes, which suited him fine. I stood by the door and watched him. When it was time to go, he ran up to me, hugged and kissed me and told me to have a good day.

I was on my way out the door when he suddenly yelled, "Mommy!" Everyone turned, half expecting him to start crying for me to return. Instead, he ran towards me and hugged and kissed me again, then ran off to re-join the others.

When I came to pick him up at the end of the day, he was busy working on another Lego™ creation that consisted of a complicated arrangement of side panels and blocks.

"It's a mosquito catcher, Mom," he explained. "The mosquito goes in here, and gets trapped in here, and we let him go out here."

I was suddenly struck by the irony of his explanation – this child, who was trying so hard to preserve all of God's tiniest creatures, was in the fight of his life. At that moment I realized that Tristan was teaching his mother that preserving life and living each moment were what life was all about.

Our family has learned to embrace these little moments, like stopping to watch ants amble across the pavement, looking at different shaped leaves, or turning over rocks to see their sparkles. We walk through the park and feed the ducks, swans and squirrels. As we feed the ducks dry pieces of bread, we try to figure out who's a girl duck and who's a boy duck, what they're quacking means, and where they sleep at night. On one particular day, a little girl was feeding the ducks and she ran out of bread. I reached into our bread bag and gave her some bread.

Tristan looked at me and said, "You're very kind, Mommy," and he reached into the bag and handed her some more bread. And I thought, that's all it takes. It's really very simple. Life is really a collection of precious moments all strung together. Getting lost in them seems to make time stand still for a while.

People say we should live for today, but I say it's not enough. We must live for the moment, because it's all we truly have. Learning to live in the moment is the most powerful lesson I have learned. You have to muscle into every moment, because every moment counts, especially knowing those moments will someday be gone.

One evening, as I lay down with Tristan in his bed, he announced that he wished God never made mosquitoes because they were always biting him. I told him that everything has a purpose, even mosquitoes.

"What's purpose?" asked Tristan.

"Purpose means that everything has a reason for being here, like mosquitoes. They're important because they feed birds."

"What's my purpose, Mommy?" he asked.

"I'm not sure, Honey. Sometimes our purpose isn't known at first, and we learn it along the way," I replied, saying the first words that sprang into my head. "Maybe your purpose is to teach people."

"What's your purpose, Mommy?" he asked.

"I don't know, Honey, but I think it's to teach also. I'm just not sure how...."

We all have a purpose, planted deep within us, something uniquely ours that we are to bring forward in this life. Finding our life's purpose is one of the dark night's greatest gifts to us, but we need to release our past ills to give the planted seed room to grow. Releasing is a necessary part of the process, which results in a different way of seeing things, like wearing new glasses, in which to view the world. It forever changes us. I was about to find my new pair of glasses in the coming years.

REAL GYM (1981)

Over the next few years, I learned everything I could about training and eating. I had outgrown my small home-made gym and I moved to a 'real' gym with real equipment. The gym was filled with local athletes – biathletes, skiers, triathletes and rock climbers – and I would eagerly watch them all from the sidelines. They used heavy weights and their execution was flawless. For these athletes, it was as if every rep was like a work of art. It was poetry in motion.

DAD (1982)

That winter, I got a call from my uncle in Ontario. My father had died from a massive heart attack while sleeping in his bed. He was 47 years old.

I was devastated. There were no last words and no chance to say good-bye. I lost trust in a Universe that could be so swift and callous in its taking. Even in his harshest moments, I knew that my father loved and cared for me deeply. I started to ponder what life was all about. Life seemed worthless and without meaning, and I felt myself drift into a grey depression. I began to feel out of control.

I started to drink away my sadness with my fellow co-workers. After the pub closed, we partied until sunrise, then we'd lock up and head out to the local diner for some breakfast. We would then disperse and go home to bed and sleep until 2 p.m. The next day we'd repeat it again, and again. Before long, four years had slipped by, and I had barely noticed. I had been anesthetised to it all.

LOVER BOY

When I was 26, I fell in love with a local boy who at one time had a promising career in sports, but he had got mixed up in drugs and lost his opportunity. He was charismatic, quick and handsome – the same qualities my father had – but unbeknownst to me, he was still addicted to alcohol and drugs, mainly crack cocaine.

One evening I caught him getting high in the living room and I was curious. He set up the pipe for me and I took a hit. From that first moment, I was addicted. It was pure euphoria. The drugs lifted me out of my grey cloud, for awhile, and I felt strangely powerful again. But the cloud always returned, and the cycle repeated itself, night after night.

That year, we spent every last penny on drugs. I was numbing myself to life, and I was operating on auto pilot, but the darkness inside of me was building up again.

I became anaemic and I started to lose my hair. My weight plummeted to 100 pounds. I hid in the house most of the time, and I only went out at night to get more 'supplies'. After a year of this, I was fired from my job, we were being evicted from our house, and in serious debt.

I had tried to quit the drugs many times, but I couldn't. They were a strong force, and one I used to numb my pain. While getting high one night, I lay back on the bed and stared at the ceiling. My heart was palpitating hard, and I struggled to breathe. I closed my eyes and wondered if it was going to end. After several minutes I opened my eyes. I was still breathing.

The next morning, I grabbed our drug paraphernalia and I went outside and smashed them into bits in the driveway, making sure to crush every last remaining pieces under my heels. Two days later, we packed up our belongings and left town.

We headed to the west coast. I hoped that a fresh start in a new city would help us get our life back in order, but it didn't work. I was staying clean, but my boyfriend wasn't. He would be gone for days at a time, and when he came home, there were more bills to pay and more debts owed. There seemed no way of escaping it. Life began to spiral down again.

MY FRONT STEPS (1989)

By now, although I was working two jobs, I couldn't get us out of debt. We had our car possessed, our dog stolen, and we were being evicted from our house. I knew our relationship was over, but I didn't know how to end it. I felt too ashamed to reach out to anyone for help, and so I stayed – and prayed that I would find a way out.

One evening, my boyfriend accused me of cheating on him, and he became furious. He punched me and threw me into the wall, and I fell into a heap on the floor. Fear washed over me, and I knew in that moment I was in real danger. I had to get away.

After he left, I sat on my front porch and looked out at the ocean. I was 29 years old and I wondered if I would live to see my 30th birthday. I called my sister and finally told her everything. The next day she sent me a plane ticket and I secretly packed up and I flew to her home up north. Fearing my boyfriend would find me and bring me home, I kept her location a secret.

My sister found me work at a local restaurant. I quickly fell into a routine of working nights and training at the local gym during the day. I struggled to understand everything that happened the last few years. I blamed myself for the breakdown in my relationship, thinking that that if I was more beautiful / loving / perfect, my boyfriend would have changed.

In time, I realized this was one of my many dysfunctional patterns of thinking from my past: where I believed that if I had been a better daughter, perhaps my parents would have loved me more. I could see that all my life I had looked for my source of self-worth and my power from other people around me. Now, I needed to find it within.

That winter, my step-mother died. She was only 41 years old. We had become distant after my father's death, and I missed her in my life, but we never created the chance to mend our differences. My real mother was living her own life, and we hadn't spoken in years. At 29 I had no parents in my life. I suddenly felt very much alone in the world.

PANIC ATTACKS

That winter, I met and fell in love with a man and we moved to Whistler, BC. He was a kind and thoughtful person, and our relationship blossomed. With his patience and support, I was able to start to feel a sense of renewed hope again. He saw the good in me, and because of this, I began to see the good in myself too. He helped me realize that

I was indeed a good person worthy of love. I needed to hear that over and over again, and he would tell me so dozens of times each day.

We rented a small apartment, and settled into our quiet mountain life. One evening, I was sitting on the bed watching TV when I felt it first hit me. It was like a giant ocean wave had come out of nowhere, and I felt dizzy and light. My heart raced and I couldn't catch my breath. My whole body was trembling. I didn't know what was happening to me. I was having a panic attack.

Over the next few days, I was riddled with more attacks. I became consumed in compulsive, repetitive rituals, like checking the stove, checking under the couch, and looking in cupboards over and over again. I felt out of control and powerless every moment. I had to quit driving, because I envisioned dragging some helpless animal under my car. I hid out in my house because I imagined my former boyfriend was hiding in the dark woods with a shotgun pointed at my head. Nothing made any sense anymore.

I had up to 30 attacks a day. I was losing touch with reality. I would call my boyfriend in the middle of an attack, and he would come home several times a day to hold me while I cried in his arms. What was happening to me? My body, once so strong and capable, was deceiving me. I felt like I was living without my skin.

THE CHOICE

I finally went to see a doctor. After a lengthy neurological assessment, she told me I had two options: take anti-anxiety drugs for life or head into counselling.

"I won't kid you," she said. "The counselling will be very, very hard work, but it will give you lasting results. It will get to the root of it all. Drugs will only mask the problem."

Presented in that manner, the choice was easy: I signed up for counselling.

She suggested a psychologist friend of hers who lived part-time in Whistler, which was the best option because I couldn't drive and it was hard for me to leave the house for any real length of time. I just had to make my way down the road a bit to her office. My boyfriend would get me there.

JANE (summer 1990)

I began working with Jane three times a week for two hours at a time. We opened up years of buried pain as I relived my father's betrayal, my step-mother's verbal and physical attacks, my mother's emotional distance, my step-father's alcoholic rages, and my own years of addiction and depression. It was raw, painful work, and at times, I wondered if I would survive.

I came to see that over the years, I had learned how to shut down. It was my way of protecting myself. I was almost 30 years of age and my spirit had had enough. My body was releasing all those damned-up memories through the panic attacks.

Now, with my body being in constant overdrive, I had to stop exercising, as any exertion would bring on another heart-pounding rush of adrenaline. Training had always been my stress reliever, but it was working against me now, and I had to give in. So I started walking instead, and I walked the mountain trails for hours, crying and listening to music in my earphones.

Month after month, with Jane's guidance, I learned to acknowledge my pain. I was learning to *speak my truth*. I was connecting with my inner self, and I was starting to see things differently now: how I took the blame for things that were not my responsibility, and how I carried the world on my shoulders. After all, I was the responsible daughter who desperately wanted her father's approval. But I was not responsible for my parents' short comings… they were never mine to own, and it was time to give them all back.

CALLING BACK MY SPIRIT

That summer was a transformative time for me. Every session, Jane and I would delve deeper and deeper into my childhood. There, in the safety and security of her office, I would hold up parts of my life, and lift them up to the sky, and let them go. Every evening I would go home and write about my days' work, and bit by bit I knit up the loose threads of my life. I was slowly calling back my spirit.

Every day as I released more pain, the panic attacks lessened bit by bit. With every release, my body began to lighten up. For the first time in years, I was sleeping soundly, and all the tension in my back and neck released. My digestion improved and I felt clear again. My ears, which had been buzzing wildly since the panic attacks started, had finally stopped ringing.

The panic attacks continued for another full year, but with Jane's guidance, I learned to not fear them. They now acted like a reminder to me of when I was headed off course, and now I could change the pattern. In time, I was able to return to exercise, but I viewed my body differently now. It had become my radio of sorts, transmitting signals to tell me when I was off frequency. I had come to respect it and I was learning how to listen, to *really* listen, to what it was trying to tell me. Body and spirit are indeed one.

Today, when I feel the first signs of panic, I stop and listen. The panic never comes. Instead, I'm able to listen and act immediately. I will forever be thankful for Jane. With her professional guidance and love, I was able to face my darkness and to release my pain. I was seeing my life through new glasses.

I had learned an important lesson, that I didn't need to own what wasn't mine. I was finally learning to give it all back. Now, being free from the weight of it all, I was ready to move forward. I was ready to get back into the land of the living, but there were still more hurdles that lay ahead of me.

FIRST CONTEST (1991)

In May, I would be turning 30 years old, and with the panic attacks behind me, my body and my mind felt strong and focused. I had returned to weight training full time, but I still needed to be careful, because too much exertion would tax my still-healing body and I would feel a wave of panic sneaking up. But I could control it now. Life was returning to *normal*.

At this point, I had been training for almost eight years and body building in Canada was still in its infancy. There was a local show coming up, so I signed up. I had nine months to prepare, so I read magazines on how to train and eat for a body building contest.

I trained six days a week, working each body part twice a week and I wrote down everything I ate. I was training for 90 minutes to 2 hours at a time, clearly too much, but I still believed that more was better, and I believed that the one who worked the longest and the hardest would succeed, a left-over belief from my childhood.

INNER SHIFTS

The training was tough, but it wasn't nearly as hard as the dieting. I was hungry and I was constantly thinking about food. I knew something had to change or I wouldn't be able to make it through the months of preparation that still lay ahead. I calculated that I needed to lose almost 30 pounds, so I decided what was needed was a change in thinking. I needed to alter my reality.

I taught myself that whenever I felt hungry, I would now see it as a positive sign that I was losing fat, so now hunger pangs were a good thing! After this inner shift, the dieting became easy. I had simply re-wired my brain!

CHANCE ENCOUNTER

During one workout, Canadian champion strength trainer Charles Poliquin was in the gym training members of the national downhill ski team. While I was doing a leg press, Charles walked over and pointed out that my left leg was over-taking the right. "Look at how your feet are sitting on the platform," he said.

The toes of my left foot were pointing out more than the toes on my right foot (an imbalance I still have to work on today).

"Focus," he said. "It's not about what you lift, it's *how* you lift. Pay attention to the little things."

I asked him about pre-contest carbohydrate foods like pasta and oatmeal, foods that most body builders steered clear of because they fear putting on weight.

"Do you eat oatmeal?" he asked.

Yes, I said.

"Then keep eating it," he said. "It obviously works for you. Everyone's different. You have to listen to your body. Most athletes don't."

It was sage advice coming from one of North America's top strength and conditioning coaches.

THIRD EYE

Before heading to bed at night, I practiced my stage routine in front of the mirror, and once in bed, I would continue practising it in my head. Going through my routine in my imagination became so real to me that I could actually hear the crowd and feel the bright lights on my skin. I felt as if I was actually up on stage!

I had done this for years with my piano recitals: I would 'play' my song on my lap in the car on the way to the theatre. In metaphysics, it's called using your third eye, or recently better known as the Law of Attraction. Now, with my posing, I was calling on that same ability.

CONTEST DAY (APRIL 21, 1991)

The day of the contest finally arrived, and we headed to the gym for the weigh-in. I had never seen a female bodybuilder in the flesh before, and now I was surrounded by them. I was very intimidated, and

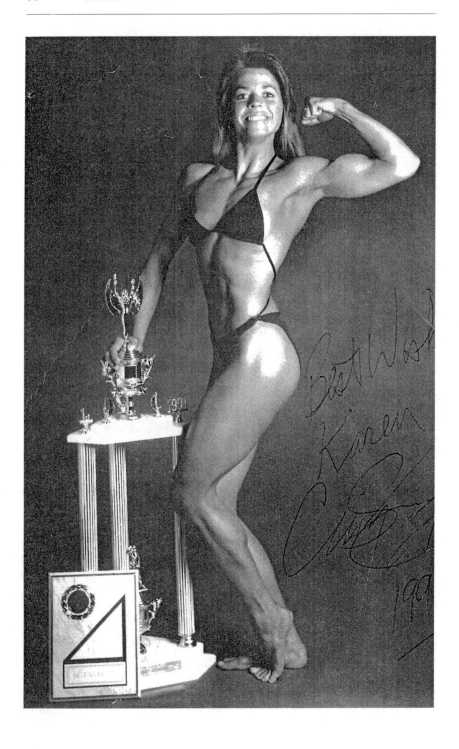

I kept my sweat suit on the entire time. I was unsure I belonged there, with those elite women.

When I finally stepped on the scale, I weighed 110 pounds. I had lost a total of 28 pounds! I had done it! I was under 114 pounds (my goal) and I would be competing as a lightweight.

That night, I went back to the hotel room and practised my routine again and again. I was afraid to eat anything for fear of gaining any weight and ruining my muscle definition, so I nibbled on small spoonfuls of cottage cheese and yogurt.

During the morning's pre-judging show, we were put through our five compulsory poses. I was nervous and very, very hungry, and it was hard to smile for the judges while trying to pose, but I gave it my all. The morning show is where you make your first impression with the judges, and they assess your muscularity, symmetry and conditioning. A competitor's placing is often determined at this show, and it can be hard to change your placing after that, but I was able to (unknowingly) move up in position between shows because I had 'carbed up' well, a tricky technique where you slowly fill up your muscles with carbohydrates over a long period of time.

The changes in my physique were astounding: the night before I appeared flat and drawn, but I sipped on a carbohydrate blend the day of the show, and by the evening show, my muscles appeared full

My first contest, the BC Gold's Classic, 1991. Having shed 28 pounds, I was now 110 pounds and 13% body fat. I won Best Lightweight and Best Overall. I weight-trained for 7 years before entering my first contest, which created greater "muscle maturity" that judges like: fuller, more defined muscle bellies with deeper, more defined cuts.

and thick, my skin was razor thin and my abs suddenly 'popped out'. Apparently all eyes were on me because of the vast difference in my physique from the morning to the evening show.

MY BAG OF ROCKS

As a parting gift, Jane had given me a small bag with three beautiful rock crystals in it. Each rock held a different energetic meaning: one banished fear, another built confidence and the third brought success. Holding them in my fist backstage reminded me of all I had been through, and I was thankful for all that Jane had taught me. After years of struggle, I was finally living my dream. I was about to step onto that stage!

As my music started, I took a deep breath and walked out. The stage lights were bright, so I just focused on finding the 'X' on centre stage. My heart was pounding and my legs were shaking. I planted my foot and made my first turn....

My routine was flawless (hadn't I practiced it a thousand times in my head?). I felt graceful and smooth, and I smiled at the judges. Even with all my years of doing piano recitals, that brief 90-second posing routine seemed like the hardest and the longest performance I had ever done.

After all the routines were done, the judges called three competitors back to the stage. I heard my name being called. Whew, I thought, I made top three! We lined up on stage beside each other, and the crowd was getting excited now. The judges called out the third place winner's name... *Not mine...* I thought. I had made the top two! They called out the second place winner... *Not me again...*

Does that mean that I won? For a moment it didn't register, then I put my hands up to my face in disbelief! I had won the Lightweight Class, my very first contest!

I walked backstage, put on my sweatsuit and grabbed my bag of rocks. A fellow competitor congratulated me and asked me what was in my bag.

"They're my power totems," I told her. "They give me strength."

"Wow," she said. "I need to get me some of those!"

Later that evening, I competed against the winners of the middle-weight and heavyweight classes and I won Best Overall! I had done what I had dreamed about in my little garage so many years ago. I had competed in my first body building contest and I was the overall winner!

At the end of the show, an old acquaintance from Banff stopped by to congratulate me. "Wow, just a few years ago, you were in a heap of trouble in Banff, and now you're out here winning body building contests!" she said. "What a difference a few years make!"

Indeed, I thought.

CLIMBING THE COMPETITION LADDER

The following year I moved to Alberta and I set my sights on the Pro-vincials. My colleagues told me I could never win a provincial contest drug-free, which motivated me even more! I asked for sponsorship from a handful of local businesses and in exchange I promised them a photo of me holding one of the top three trophies. They asked me how I was so sure I could come in top three. "I just know," I told them.

I headed first to the regionals, and I again won the Lightweight

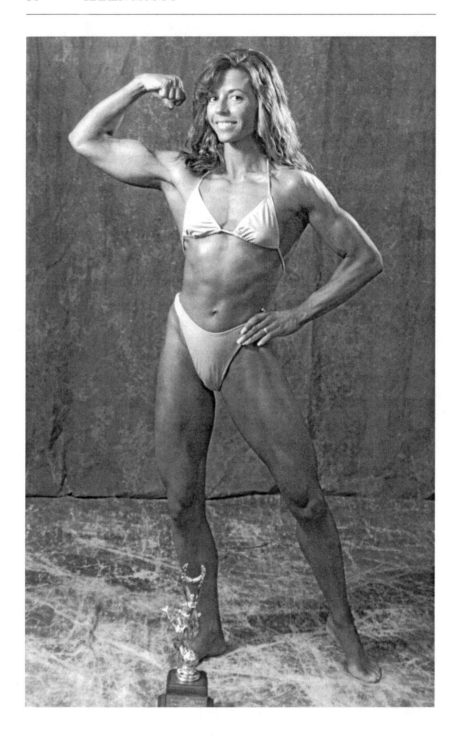

Class but I missed out on Best Overall. The winner was smaller and softer, but she had stage presence to die for! I was told I had the better physique, but when we went on stage, she outshone me. It was a valuable lesson to learn – confidence sells and clearly I still needed to work on mine.

Two weeks later, I competed at the Provincials. Trying to keep your 'peak' with two contests so close together is challenging, and I was competing against several women who were known steroid users and whose bodies were packed with hard, thick muscle. It was a tough battle, and I gave it my all. I wasn't sure of my chances, but I knew I had put everything I had into my training and preparation. In the end, the judges awarded me the Lightweight Winner and I went on to win Best Overall! I was now a Provincial Body Building Champion!

According to the judges, my superb conditioning and my feminine lines were what won them over. The judges were admittedly trying to stem the tide of drugs coming into the sport now, and as one judge put it, "We want to keep our women *women*." I had the right look and the right level of conditioning at the right time. It was a valuable lesson in fortitude, and that not all wins are based on size. Quality over quantity.

I had done the impossible. I had won a provincial contest drug-

---

I won the Southern Albertans Lightweight class, and 2 weeks later I won Best Overall at the Alberta Provincials. Many said I could never win a provincial contest drug-free, but I proved it could be done! That was a tough win because I had to hold my peak conditioning for 2 long weeks between shows!

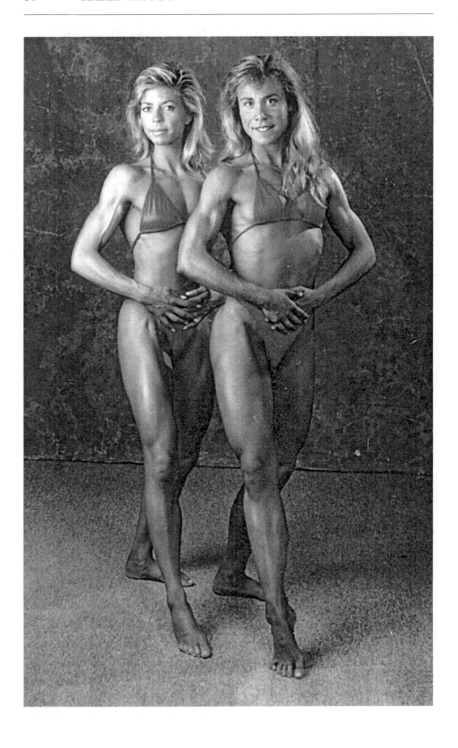

free, something that was a rarity back then (and still rare today). The following week I delivered a picture of me holding my first place trophy to all my sponsors.

A PAINFUL LOSS

The following year, I decided to go back to college. Body building was a great sport and I loved it, but I knew deep down that it was unlikely I would be able to make a living at it. I decided to enroll in a recreation program, to blend my love of sports with the great outdoors.

I loved being back in school, and it was an incredibly stimulating and exciting time for me. I threw myself into my studies. I became an honour student and I received a partial scholarship.

I trained at a nearby gym with another woman, Jacquie, who was a former triathlete who wanted me to train her for her first body building show. I created a triple split program for us and we trained five days a week together. I welcomed the company. It was nice to have a fellow female to train with, and someone who was as diligent and as hard-working as me.

After eight months of steady training, we set our sights on the Western Canadian Body Building Show, the second highest show in the country. We packed our car and drove to the weigh-in.

Me and friend Jacqueline Lewis at the Western Canadians in 1994. I was second place Lightweight, and I trained Jacquie who came in third in Heavyweight, a good placing for her first competition. Being a lifelong athlete, Jacquie was a dream to coach because she had a lot of passion for training. After this contest, she went on to become a member of the Canadian Triathlon Team for 10 years.

NO STEROIDS

At the show, I learned that I would be competing against an old rival (one whom I had previously beaten) who had started taking steroids. She was now a solid ten pounds heavier (and with an altered face and voice), and I didn't stand a chance. She was awarded first place and I placed second.

I was heartbroken. I knew I had trained just as hard, and we had the same body type and level of conditioning, but she simply out-muscled me pound for pound. Clearly, at this level of competition, the judges were saying that size did indeed matter. It was a tough loss.

I pondered my future. I had never considered taking drugs because I only ever wanted to compete clean and fair. I wanted to honour my body in all ways, and I had struggled to regain my health after years of substance abuse and panic attacks, so I wasn't about to jeopardize my health again. I also knew that taking steroids would mean I would have to lie to family and friends, and I couldn't live with that. I wanted to live honestly. I wanted to live in my truth, because I'd learned that if I didn't, my health would suffer. I had suffered enough.

PREGNANT

After the Westerns, I hung up my weight training belt and we moved to a small town in BC near the ocean. We bought a small home and soon afterward, we were married. We decided we wanted to have a child, but I was concerned that my many years of low body fat would hamper our efforts. However, once I started eating normally and my body fat went up to a healthy 20%, we conceived quickly. In March, the ultrasound showed I was carrying a boy!

For the rest of the pregnancy, I had terrible morning sickness. All I could eat were sugary carbohydrates like cereal, muffins and crackers which left me feeling bloated and depressed. My energy plummeted and I felt depressed. I was shaky and sick all the time, so I had to stop training altogether.

Admittedly, it was hard for me to watch my baby-body develop. I watched my belly expand in ways I never could have imagined. Just a year ago I was competing on stage with a rock-hard body. Now that body was barely recognizable underneath my newly acquired mommy-flesh. It was all just a distant memory now.

TRISTAN'S BIRTH (December 30, 1995)

After three days of hard labour, Tristan was delivered by caesarian section on December 30th, 1995. He appeared to be a healthy, happy baby with no outward signs of any trouble. He had an abnormally slow heart beat, which I assumed was genetic because I had a lower heart rate also, and they put him on a heart monitor machine for several days. (We found out years later that this is one of the signs of DMD.)

I was so unsure of what to do as a new mother. I never felt like I had a strong, caring and reliant mother figure in my life, so I had no role model to draw from. I felt clumsy and awkward, and I cried most days. A cloud had descended over my life.

The following year, we moved to the Interior of BC. I was sad to leave my beloved ocean, and I continued to feel lost in the challenges of motherhood. Once we settled down, I decided I needed to find something satisfying, something that I could work on over time and that I could call my own. I needed to get plugged back in, so I checked out the local university.

I signed up for the journalism program. I always loved writing, and a journalism degree offered a more definite career path. My college recreation diploma helped fill the program's first and second year of prerequisites, so I could fast track and complete my degree in two years. I started classes that fall.

DIVORCE (1998)

I immediately immersed myself in my studies. I loved the program, and I loved learning again. I was surrounded by like-minded people, and I enjoyed the camaraderie and support of this growing, active and educated group.

The stress of our move, buying a new home, and a new baby, was putting an immense strain on our marriage, and we now had my schooling to contend with. My husband wanted me to work, and I wanted to complete my studies. We had discussed this before we decided to get pregnant but now the goal posts had been moved. I felt betrayed and angry.

By the following year, the strain proved too much for our marriage. When Tristan was 2-1/2 years old, we filed for divorce. It was a dark and painful time for us all.

After our divorce, I continued with my studies. As a single parent, I managed to secure a small student loan to see us through. I was running on little sleep, but I felt free for the first time in years. It was like a huge weight had suddenly been lifted off my shoulders. I felt scared but excited at the same time.

Tristan and I stayed living in the house and his father moved a few doors away. I qualified for subsidized child care, so with Tristan in day care, I was able to train between classes. I was determined to shed my pregnancy fat and get my energy back. Being surrounded by dumbbells and barbells again felt good. So, with program in hand, I began to rebuild my body, again....

GOING DEEPER

After my divorce, I felt lonely but strangely liberated. I was reconnecting to my creativity and my power through my weight training and my writing. Lifting and writing were both near and dear to my heart, and I knew that they would always be important in my life, yet I was still unsure of what I was supposed to do with my life. I was still in limbo.

After many challenging years, the veil had been lifted and I was seeing and living from a different place now. My world had expanded, and I hoped that I was finally stepping into the light.

However, I was about to learn that it was going to get a whole lot darker. In fact, my journey, the *real* journey, had only just begun.

THREE

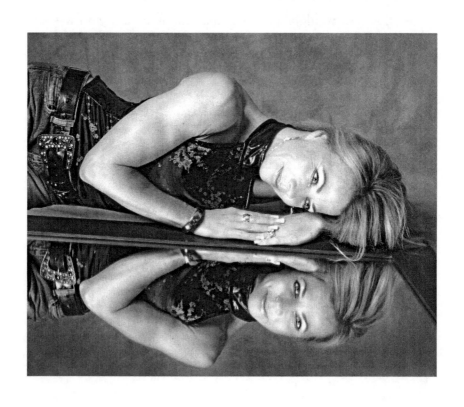

A Fall from Grace:
Body as Teacher (1999 – 2001)

THE WEDDING, WAR AND FRANK SINATRA,
OCTOBER 7, 2001 (5 months after diagnosis)

It's October 7th and I'm standing in the rain, crying. My husband and I flew out to Vancouver to attend a friend's wedding. Over 100 people arrived at this exclusive clubhouse in celebration of their union. But underneath the pink icing and bubble confetti is another reality – our friend's father is dying of cancer and they hope he will make it through the evening to see his son wed. On this same evening, the United States has declared war on Afghanistan.

I'm outside on the patio, looking out over the soft, green lawns and I marvel at how peaceful everything looks. I cried through the wedding vows, not out of joy, but because the emotion of the moment stirred up other emotions deep inside me. I cried for my friend's dying father, for the injustices of war, and for my son who may never experience the joy of marriage. Inside, Frank Sinatra's My Way *booms through the club-house halls. It was my father's favourite song and I cry some more.*

All of this reminds me that life is a precarious thing. Lately, I have found comfort in the grief of others, because it makes me feel less alone in my own grief. Suddenly, I wasn't alone in my grief because the attacks on the World Trade Centre had created a grief greater than mine, and it eased my own pain. I was experiencing schaden-freude, *a natural human reaction which refers to the embarrassing spasm of gratitude we feel when something bad happens to someone else instead of us. It makes us feel strangely safe, like when you hear of a family involved in a terrible accident, and you go home to your family and say, "We can't complain, did you hear about so-and-so who died in that awful accident?"*

With my son's diagnosis, my family had become 'that family', the one everyone measured their luck by. It was a yardstick I didn't want to own, but was to be played out for many years to come.

The terrorist attacks created a public grief, but my grief remains a private one. While strangers all over the world reach out to victims of terrorism, I am hard-pressed to get a neighbour to cross the street to see how we are doing. When my husband took a job up north for the winter, I thought, "surely our neighbours would come and help me shovel the driveway, or see how we're doing." No one came. I felt confused and angry.

"Why won't they reach out to help us?" I often asked my husband. "They know about Tristan, don't they care?" It would be some time before I understood their silence.

Several months later I was watching a show on the families of vic-tims lost in the September 11th attacks. A well-known TV psychologist was urging the family of one distraught woman, whose husband had died, to not pull away from her. "Often times when we say, "Oh, I went to visit so-and-so today and she's doing much better," what we're really saying is, "She didn't make me feel uncomfortable today." It lets us off the hook." Now I understood. My son's diagnosis made people uncomfortable. We had become a reminder of what could happen when you're looking the other way.

I'm learning to settle my anger, but it's a slow process. Our family's struggle with muscular dystrophy has caused a sifting out of people to one side or the other. On one side are people who stay tight within themselves. I am learning to let them go with love. On the other side are the people who offer help without being asked, who want to learn everything they can about the disease, and who want to know what their role will be. They listen to our story, and when I scream, they know my anger is not directed at them, but is rather a mother's anguish at losing her only child.

Out on the patio, the rain continues to gently fall. Inside, Frank Sinatra is singing Dad's song. I start to cry. I miss him. I wish he could wrap his arms around me and tell me everything was going to be alright.

In times of need, we often reach outside ourselves for answers. But in doing so, we are disabling our most valuable asset – our inner guidance. As I overcame my toxic childhood, my addictions, the panic attacks and my divorce, the lessons continued to come through that most treasured of things – my body. But there were no rewards forthcoming.

I would soon move further into the darkness with the news of our son's condition, and my body would continue to carry the brunt of it all in unimaginable and painful ways.

AT THE SCREEN DOOR (1999)

After my divorce, the bills started piling up, so I took on extra work as a freelance writer. My small student loan was helping us keep our heads above water, but it was running out fast.

For the next year, I slept very little, relying on coffee and adrenaline to keep me going. Friends told me that I should quit college and move in with family. I was furious. My ex's life (and work) continued after divorce, why couldn't mine? I was not about to abandon my dream of getting a degree, and I would finish, no matter what.

Our daily routine was always the same: drop Tristan off at day care, go to classes, train at the gym during lunch, do some freelance work, pick up Tristan, drive home, have dinner, read a book and go to bed. At bedtime, I would lay down with Tristan in his bed, being careful not to fall asleep myself. Then once he was asleep, I would head back into my office and continue working until after midnight. I would head off to bed and set the alarm for 4:30 a.m. so I could squeeze in a few more hours of work before Tristan woke up.

My crazy schedule was catching up with me. My body constantly trembled, and I wasn't able to hold any food down. My weight dropped to 103 pounds and my body ached all the time. My doctor suggested I take anti-depressants, which I declined. I wasn't depressed, I was just worn out. With no family support and with the bills constantly piling up, I wondered how we would make it through.

One morning, while I was standing at the screen door getting ready to leave, my whole body started to tremble. I squeezed my hands together tight trying to stop the shaking. I closed my eyes, took a deep breath and said quietly, "Please, Universe, help me through just one more day. Just one more day, *please.*"

MY WATERFALL

On weekends, I would grab Tristan and we would walk up to a small waterfall located behind our house. Few people knew about the waterfall, and it became our little get-away during hot summer days. It was our private place, and we would sit and throw rocks into the swirling waters. I felt peaceful sitting there, and I would often say a silent prayer to the waterfall. I didn't know how we were going to get through, but I had faith that somehow, some way, it would all work out.

ARMS WIDE OPEN

After one particularly tough week, I packed up Tristan and we headed to the waterfall. I was exhausted and fed up, and I desperately needed an end to our struggles. Once there, I stood at the edge of the falls, threw my arms open, looked up to the sky and shouted, "Now what?" I was tired of struggling and I needed some answers. I did it again and again, each time shouting louder, "NOW WHAT?"

In that moment, I gained another little piece of the puzzle: I was learning the importance of surrender. For that moment in time, my body and my mind no longer felt closed off and tight. It was like I became *unstuck*. In that moment, with arms flung open wide, I had made an important shift in my healing with this newest skill of mine.

I have taught this little lesson to thousands of women over the years with profound results. Our body and our mind are a mirror reflection of each other, and when we close down our bodies, our minds are closed also. Physically opening ourselves up to our journey, good or bad, and saying yes to our struggles with *arms wide open* helps us move forward.

That fall, I was offered a full-time freelance position with a small company, and I gladly accepted. I would be able to earn more money for Tristan and me, and hopefully be able to pay off some bills.

CHERYL

One day, a colleague had just returned from a tarot card reading with a visiting psychic. I had played with tarot cards in the past, and I was always intrigued by them, so I called to book an appointment. The psychic had an opening the next day. I was apprehensive, but I promised myself to stay open to all possibilities. At this point in my life, I had nothing to lose.

When I first met Cheryl, I was impressed by her professionalism and her *normalness*. She was engaging, funny and *real*.

"What I do is a skill, like anything else," she explained. "Everyone has the ability, some more than others. I just happened to be born with it."

She shuffled the deck and explained the process to me. She said psychics don't really predict the future, rather, they can tell you the future *if you maintain the path you are on*. As humans, we are always free to alter it.

"We are co-creators of our world," she explained. "Our life is not all mapped out for us. We always have free will and choice to change it at any time."

For the next hour, she revealed my past with incredible accuracy. I learned that I was an *empathic*, meaning I felt things more than others, like colours, scents, music and other people's emotions. This explained how, as a child, I could amaze my family with my 'seeing' ability: I would grab coloured balls, close my eyes, rub the balls, and tell them what colour each was because I could 'feel' the colour in my hand. It also explained why I felt uncomfortable in crowds, why certain fabrics would unhinge me, and why certain paint colours made me feel uneasy.

This also explained my affinity for water, because water helps to cleanse and balance the empathic person's sensitive and sometimes highly-charged nervous system.

"Whether you're in it or on it, you need the cleansing properties of water. You always have," said Cheryl. She also explained that being an empathic meant that my lessons – my intuition and my guidance – would always come through my body. "In particular, the *nervous system*," she said.

I needed to be careful of this, and it would benefit me to learn its language so I could better use these unique tools in my life.

MY PURPOSE

During the reading, I asked her if Tristan and I were going to be okay.

"You will be more than okay," she said. "Everyone brings forward something in this life. It's like a job we are here to do on Earth. For some it's creating beautiful music, for others it's math, and for still others it's science."

Then she looked straight at me and said, "You're life's purpose is inspiration. You're here *to inspire*."

How could that be? I certainly didn't feel like I could inspire anyone, let alone myself most days. I was broke and tired, but I was here to inspire others? It just didn't make sense to me. She continued with her reading.

She described Tristan: "You knew him before he was born. You've had him in previous lives, and always in the closest of relationships. He's been with you for all your lifetimes."

I asked her to describe him to me as she saw him. She described a tall athletic young man, with dark hair and dark eyes, and he was dressed in a T-shirt and dark pants. I felt a shiver go up my spine: this was the same young man who had visited my dreams for years, and who I would see off in the distance.

"Your son was your brother in your last life," she explained, "and in that life, he looked after you. You promised him that you would return the favour in the next life time. Now it's your turn to look out for him."

I asked what Tristan's purpose was.

"He has a way with animals, always has. This is a child of the future and he comes with ideas and thoughts that will be put into use well into the future."

Her reading gave me strength and comfort, and I came to understand that our lives are in perfect working order, and that Tristan and I were somehow a part of that divine order.

CHAKRAS AND AURAS

That summer, things began to shift for me. It was like I had stepped through a portal and I began to experience new kinds of energy. I felt strange sensations in my body, like a breeze inside of me. It was like someone put a hollow pipe inside my spine, and I could sense warm air running through it, and I could 'see' colours at various points along the pipe. (I hadn't learned anything about the chakra system at this point, but I suspect this was what I was experiencing.)

At dusk, I was able to see bluish shadows around trees and plants. (Again, I hadn't learned about auras yet, but likely this is what I was experiencing.) I was feeling a kind of connectedness with my surroundings, like a giant invisible web had been thrown over everything, and everything was connected to everything else.

Something had been awakened in me.

THE CAMPFIRE

One evening after I put Tristan to bed, I went out to my campfire and I sat down and began to write. In a class, Cheryl taught us that we were all co-creators of our world, and with focus and intention we could manifest our desires. So with pen in hand, I began to write out my wish-list of what I wanted in a mate.

I wrote down all the things I wanted in a partner including his level of education, his body-type, his choice of work, and I even saw him with several dogs. I also wanted someone who had been married but who had no children, and someone who loved the outdoors. And he had to drive a truck!

I closed my eyes and went through each of my points, focusing in and *feeling* them as if they were already present in my life. I knew that the key to manifesting anything was to feel as if it was already a reality. I repeated this exercise every night for two weeks. Then I tucked my journal away.

Six months later, my future husband (and his two dogs!) walked into my life. We fell madly in love, and we spent every waking hour together. Finally, I had someone to love and share my life with. It would be years before I would pull out those original writings again, and I would be amazed at what I would find – he had every one of qualities I had listed!

They say the Universe always gives you what you ask for. In my case, it certainly did. I was hooked into something greater than myself, an energy source that I would learn to call on as the journey got deeper.

LOSS

I now had a partner to share my life with, and I was thankful for the added support. My financial worries were now over, but being in a partnership brought up old issues for me, and I found myself struggling again with what a woman's role was supposed to be – lesser of a bread winner and more of a homemaker – and I rallied against the unspoken ways of the world. We also differed widely in our parenting views, and at times tempers flared, but we were determined to make our union work.

We wanted to build our family so we decided to have a baby. Within two months, I was pregnant but several months later, we lost our baby. Six months later, I became pregnant again, but again I miscarried. We were devastated.

We poured ourselves into our collective life and tried to heal. I completed my journalism degree, and shortly after graduation, I took a job as a reporter at the local newspaper. I was finally making a living with my writing, and I loved my work. My partner and I kept busy with our respective work and with raising Tristan, and in time, we were slowly able to put our losses behind us.

CITY MOVE (2000)

It was the New Millennium and we wanted a fresh start, so we decided to move to Ottawa. I didn't want to leave our mountain home, but it was a good work opportunity for my partner. His family all lived there, so Tristan and I would be able to meet his family for the first time and get to know them.

We rented a small house in the heart of the city and settled in. My partner's job was up north, so he flew home every second weekend. I felt lonely without him, and I struggled to fit into my new city life. It seemed like the city never slept! There were the constant sounds of honking horns, music blaring and there were people everywhere! I felt rattled all the time. I missed the quietness of my old home out west and I longed to be back there.

That spring, I became pregnant for a third time and we were cautiously optimistic, but again, three months into the pregnancy, we lost the baby. I was still weak from the other miscarriages, and I struggled to regain my strength. I was tired all the time and I couldn't shake the constant feeling of uneasiness.

I didn't feel comfortable confiding to my partner's family about how I was feeling, so I kept everything to myself. I felt depressed and lonely, and I felt like I just didn't fit in anywhere. By now, Tristan was in kindergarten for a few hours every day, so with some free time during the day, I signed up at a nearby gym.

It was my first workout in many months, and after several minutes, I noticed something just wasn't right. I felt unusually tired and my body felt strange. I left the gym after only training for 20 minutes. The next day, my joints felt tight, and my body seemed to be vibrating. My fingertips and my toes started to tingle, and I had a constant headache. The strange body sensations never left.

Week after week, my symptoms got worse, and I eventually stopped going to the gym. The one thing that I loved and that always helped me through – my training – was not helping me anymore. What was happening to me?

I went to see several doctors. They ran countless tests on me, and they checked me for a host of diseases including ALS, multiple sclerosis, heart or neurological issues and cancer but everything showed up negative. One doctor prescribed anti-depressants to me, and I refused them. I told him I wasn't sick in body, but that my spirit was hurting. I told him that I hated the city, I felt rattled all the time, and my body and my mind felt like they were constantly 'turned on'. There was no peaceful place for me anywhere.

He looked at me with a blank look on his face and handed me the prescription for anti-depressants. I walked out, tossing it into the garbage can. I would find my own way to heal myself.

TRISTAN'S DIAGNOSIS (May 21, 2001)

That spring, I made a doctor's appointment for Tristan. His teacher commented that he didn't seem as strong as the other boys, and we noticed he had started to walk with a strange step, so we assumed the problem was in his hips. Just a few weeks prior, we had enrolled him in soccer camp, and we noticed how differently he ran from the other boys. (We didn't have any other children of our own to relate him to.) He had always been small for his age, though we thought that with time he would catch up.

The paediatrician sent us to a specialist at Children's Hospital and once there, our son went for blood tests. On May 19th, 2001, our son was diagnosed with Duchenne Muscular Dystrophy (DMD).

DMD is a fast progressing, degenerative disease that affects boys (there are only a few reported cases of it happening to girls). Due to a mutation, there is a tail missing on the 'X' chromosome, and so with the DNA (genetic code) now broken, the body is therefore unable to continue on with its life-long job of building and repairing muscle. The result is a slow breakdown of all the body's muscles, starting with the legs. Eventually the person loses use of their arms and hands, and they can no longer hold themselves up. The organs weaken also (because they too are muscle), including the heart and lungs.

Historically, DMD was an inherited genetic mutation, but there was no such disease in either of our families. Our son's condition was a 'spontaneous mutation'. It was a fluke accident that can happen to anyone. To date, there is no remission and there are no cures for DMD.

This explained a lot of things to us, including our son's low heart rate after birth, his late start at walking (he only started to walk at 18 months), and his poor showing at any sports we enrolled him in. It also explained how he stood and walked, with his feet further apart, as he tried to balance himself better.

It also explained his large calf muscles, which is a classic sign of DMD. People would stop me on the street and comment on his huge, shapely calves and how he had all the makings of a future body builder. *Perhaps he will follow in his mother's footsteps, they would often say.*

NIGHT WALKS

From that moment on, life as we knew it was over. Nothing seemed real anymore. It felt like we were living in a thick fog, and everything seemed to move painfully slow. We were headed into uncharted territory, and we had no idea how to move through it. There was no one to reach out to, no one who could relate to what we were going through.

I would lie awake at night crying into the darkness. When I couldn't sleep, I would throw on my hiking boots and head into the dark woods. I've always felt the safest outdoors and far away from everything and everyone, and so I walked the trails of the city's outskirts for hours on end.

I would return home just before daylight, take off my boots and head into my office and search the Internet for anything I could read about DMD. The more I read, the more desperate I became. DMD was one of the oldest recorded diseases, dating back to the 1800s, and nothing had any effect on changing the course of the disease. Ours was a disease without hope.

VISITS

We were now in the revolving door of the medical system as we visited one specialist after another. I made a promise to myself to never let Tristan see me cry, and I tried desperately to keep my sadness from him. So when I felt a wave of sadness welling up inside me, I would head into the bathroom, close the door, put a towel over my mouth and scream and cry into the towel. He never heard a thing.

Tristan was starting to ask why he had to see so many doctors. We explained to him that he was born with something called DMD, and that there were thousands of other boys with it. We told him that this was why he couldn't run as fast as the other boys. We explained that there was no cure – yet – but that doctors were always working to find something, and we hoped one day they would create a medicine to make it go away. Tristan seemed satisfied with our answers for the time being, but I knew eventually he would be asking more questions. I wasn't sure I was ready for that.

Over the next few months, Tristan's health seemed to stabilize, but now we were hyper-vigilant to every move he made. Every minor misstep or dropped toy sent us into a panic and we wondered if this was the start of it all. We didn't know what to expect or what to do. There was nothing we could do but sit and wait.

BODY PAIN

The pain in my body escalated, and my back, from skull to tailbone, was entirely seized up. My muscles felt thick and heavy, like cement and I had shooting pains in every one of my joints. I couldn't eat or sleep and I couldn't carry on a normal conversation. Talking about the weather to passer-bys seemed so frivolous and unimportant. Everyone seemed to be living on the surface, while I lived somewhere else. I longed for someone to ask me how we were, *how we truly were*, and to want to listen to the awful truth of it all – the sleepless nights, the constant fear and the never-ending sadness. But no one asked, and I felt alone in our grief. I withdrew inside myself.

At night, I kept a bottle of Tylenol by my bedside table, and I would take two pills every few hours to try to ease my pain, but it didn't help. Eventually, I would get up, slip on my boots and go walking, again. There, in the dark woods, I could lose myself, if only for awhile.

My skin constantly felt like it was on fire, and my arms and legs vibrated all the time now, like there was an electrical current shooting through them. I was shaking and I couldn't hold down food. All my tendons and ligaments seemed like they were pulled as tight as guitar strings, and my body felt hard and unyielding. If anyone touched me – anywhere – I would wince in pain. I felt like a human pin cushion. My body had become a stranger to me.

My head was filled with never-ending questions, and I felt like I was drowning in it all. I was constantly thinking about the future, and my mind was going round and round in circles, asking questions that had no answers. When would our son go into a wheelchair? When would he be unable to feed himself? Would he ever drive? Would he graduate? Would he ever get married? Could he ever have children? Would he be in pain? Who would help us?

Day after day, I kept going to the gym to train. It was all about function now, not form. *I have to stay strong for Tristan*, I thought, I have to keep this up. But I couldn't. My body was used up. Its energy supply had finally run out. In metaphysical terms, I had become energetically ill. There was nothing left of me.

Body and spirit were both broken. I would not be able to train again for six long years.

MY DIAGNOSIS

After three months, I was diagnosed with chronic fatigue syndrome and fibromyalgia, which (in my view) meant that they used the convenience of these newly-coined diseases to put a label on my symptoms. I was prescribed an eating and vitamin regime that was all too familiar to me: clean food, no man-made products, no alcohol or sugar, high quality protein and a full-out supplement regime. As a competitive athlete I had been eating this way for years. Funny, I thought, I was doing all the right stuff all along, and *I was at the pinnacle of physical strength, but even that didn't save me.*

Occasionally, I would head back to the gym to test the training waters. I had hoped that training would help loosen my chronically tight body, but it was no use. Regardless of what part of my body I trained, my whole body would tighten in response. I tried acupuncture, chiropractic work, massage and Rolfing, but nothing relieved the tension. My body was in lock-down mode.

During one massage session, the therapist placed his hands on the small rhomboid muscles of the shoulder blade area, which he was trying to relax with massage. I felt my whole body rock back and forth.

"I can't do anything for you," he finally said. "I can't even work on individual muscles to get them to loosen. It's like all your muscles have melted into one big muscle. Your entire body is locked together. I've never actually seen anything like this before."

There seemed no way out of the vicious cycle.

SHOWING SIGNS (2002)

Tristan had started walking on his toes more because his Achilles tendons were starting to shorten, a by-product of the disease. He was tripping more and he was becoming more frustrated, but we would blame it on a stick or rock that had mysteriously gotten in his way.

Stairs were becoming hard for Tristan, so we had to carry him up and down them now, and we had to lift him in and out of vehicles. We didn't walk to the beach much anymore, because it was too hard for him to walk the uneven, rocky ground. He couldn't do long walks, so we would put him in his stroller instead. People started to comment that he seemed too old to be riding in a stroller, but I never explained.

HEALERS

With doctors having little to offer us, I turned to my metaphysical roots for answers. I started taking Tristan to a host of healers, including Shamans and psychics. Nothing in his situation ever changed, yet I found comfort in alternative perspectives on disease, dying and death. We delved into crystal therapies, chakra readings, Reiki work, palmistry and iridology, and I started to see his disease outside of its genetic make-up. Perhaps there was a higher purpose to it all. Yet at the root of it was still my desperate attempt to find a cure for my son.

It was at one of these appointments when one healer, a body reader, turned to me and said, "Your job is not to save your son. Your job is to love him. As long as you're *out there* trying to save him, you're not here, really present, with him, loving him."

He was right. In my desperation, I was losing precious time with my son.

Over the next few months, I began to read everything I could by a host of New Thought authors, in order to better understand Tristan's journey. I had abandoned my desperate attempts to find a cure, but I needed to make peace and find meaning and purpose in what we were living through. I read books by Thomas Moore, Eckhart Tolle, Neale Donald Walsh, Louise Hay, Deepak Chopra, Elizabeth Kubler-Ross and Carolyn Myss. I mediated and prayed, I wrote and I cried. And I continued with my night walks.

FLUSHING PILLS

I was unable to shake my depression and sadness, and my partner begged me to find help. So I went to see a psychiatrist. After our first session, she prescribed anti-depressants for me. I protested, but she said she would not continue our work together unless I agreed to take them. "Think of them as your little angels," she said.

When I got home, I took one, and the rest of the evening I sat on the back step in a stupor. I felt lifeless. I couldn't even cry. That evening, I flushed the pills down the toilet. I needed to feel my journey, every awful step of it, not deaden myself to it. I wanted to honour Tristan and stay open to it all. I wasn't afraid.

The next day, I told her I wouldn't take any more of her 'little angels.' "I'm not crazy," I said. "I'm just really, really sad. I'm not afraid of the sadness. I need to feel it. It's okay. I can do this."

"Then I can't treat you if you don't do as I wish," she said.

I told her that was fine, and that I had already decided to fire *her*. I had a personal creed I lived by, and that included staying present to my pain. How could I make any real change if I was numbing myself to it all?

In the end, I believe it was her fear – not mine – that caused us to part ways. I was willing to go through my pain, but she was not. It was our last session together.

CONSTANT CHANGE

That year was the most painful year of my life. Day after day, I struggled with coming to terms with my son's diagnosis and all that it meant. Our son was showing more signs of progression. He had to grab onto furniture to pull himself up from the floor, and he was tripping more often. He needed to be lifted in and out of bed, and on and off the toilet. He couldn't turn on taps or turn door knobs by himself anymore.

Tristan and I at the beach. He had to be watched carefully now, because his legs were becoming increasingly weak and he would often fall down, as the DMD progressed. It was tough and painful time for all of us.

Play dates were different now: I often had to stay with Tristan while he played with his friends because he had to be carried up and down the stairs, and I needed to help him in the bathroom. If the kids were playing running or climbing games, Tristan had to sit on the sidelines and watch.

In our world, change was our only constant, and we struggled to learn how to work with this ever-moving and unpredictable new force in our lives.

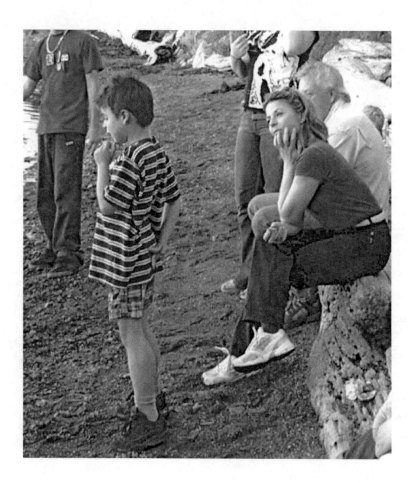

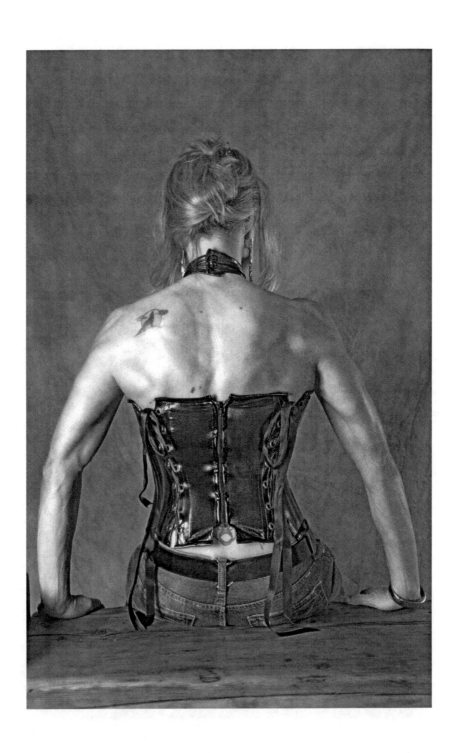

FOUR

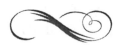

Holding On:
Wheelchairs & Crystal Balls
(2000 – 2008)

THE MUSTARD SEED, DECEMBER 15, 2001
(7 months after diagnosis)

There is a Buddhist story of a woman whose child fell ill and died. Distraught, the mother carried her child's lifeless body to the Buddha to ask for help. The Buddha told her to go into the village and collect a mustard seed from every house where no one had died. The woman obeyed, but after several days she returned with no mustard seeds. She then understood the lesson the Buddha was trying to teach her, that every family experiences death. From this lesson, she was able to accept her child's death and move forward.

When I was a young girl, death terrified me. As I grew older, I buried my fear in my school studies and work, but there was always this little tug on my heart. My first real experience with death was when my father died suddenly at the age of 47. I was 21 years old and devastated at losing my mentor, my father. I recall every detail. The endless rain, stroking my dad's cold hands and face as he lay in the casket, and watching the casket being lowered into the black earth. It was then that I became fearful of God and death. My biggest fear, that I would lose my dad, had become a reality. It was like God went inside my head and heard my deepest fear.

When doctors told me my son would die before his 21st birthday, my fears of death resurfaced. I knew I had to come to terms with death or I would be of no use to my son. I began to read books on the subject. I began talking to other people and to watch their experiences. I went on a quest of all things spiritual. I traveled to places deep within myself, where silence and truth reside, and I soon began to create a healthy relationship with death. I soon learned that I had to give up some things – my expectations of what 'normal' means – and replace it with a different understanding.

Zen hospice worker Frank Ostaseski says we should not wait for death to knock on our door before we learn the lessons it has to teach us. "Invite death in for a cup of tea. Use death as an advisor."

Other spiritual leaders, including Elisabeth Kubler-Ross and Carlos Casteneda, urge us to see death as an ally, a kind of spiritual counsel that can help us live a full life. Author Eckhart Tolle says that while many of us don't want to think about death, we're supposed to think about it. "The secret to life is to 'die before you die' – and find that there is no death."

I believe in what Gary Zukav teaches in The Seat of the Soul *that sometimes guidance must come through personal crisis, which awakens us to the potential of the soul. I am being awakened to this po-*

tential, and after a lifetime of questioning death, I am learning to sit with it awhile, and I'm getting comfortable with its presence.

In Buddhism, they say the root of all suffering is attachment. I had created an attachment to Tristan's future. I believed that my son would live a 'normal' life – marry, have children, have a career etc., but with his diagnosis, I have to alter my expectations of my son's life. I have to let go of all the things we often take for granted and replace them with a new reality.

I ask myself several important questions – "What if we were all wheelchair-bound by 12 years old? What if we all lived no longer than 21 years of age? How would 'normal' look then?" Through asking these questions, I am starting to experience a break from traditional thought. I am beginning to see with fresh eyes. I am beginning to re-create a different vision for Tristan's future, but fear and sadness still engulf me.

This letting go process continues to be a long, hard lesson. I want to hold on tight, to control the outcome and to make it right, the way it's supposed to be. But I know that with every little bit of letting go, it frees up room at the other end for something else, something better, to move in. But I cannot let go. I'm afraid to let go.

A famous actress was once asked about her secret to living a good life. Was it money? A certain acting role? Social status? Being in love?

To her it was none of those things. Having survived a tough childhood, she said simply: *"The secret to life is learning to endure."*

I understood. In my life, my ability to survive was my greatest strength. I too had learned to endure, but it's an often overlooked, yet a necessary part of the journey.

Society sees all pain as bad. We are supposed to move through it as quickly as possible – extinguish the pain – with drugs, therapy, work – and move on. Don't be a victim. Don't wallow in it. Don't drag others down with your story.

Sometimes, when we simply cannot move forward, there's wisdom in knowing that it's best to sit and hold until the storm passes, and in the midst of my son's diagnosis and my own declining health, I too was learning how to just hold my ground, for however long it took, as our storm continued to rage all around us.

RETURNING TO THE OCEAN (2002)

It had been two years since we moved to the city and it had proved to be too much for me. The endless noise and crowds of people over-stimulated my sensitive nervous system, and my body was constantly on high alert. I simply could not improve in this place. So, the following year we returned to the coast and my healing ocean.

We found a quiet, wooded lot where we could build an accessible home for Tristan. We had to consider his changing future needs in designing our house, carefully thinking through every detail. That fall, we moved into our new home. I felt more at ease, knowing we were finally settled, and I was thankful to be living in the country once again, but I would learn that I would need more than a relocation to mend myself.

MORE SIGNS

Tristan was now seven years old, and he was in grade one. His easy nature was a blessing, given all he was going through, and he seemed to take most things in stride. He had a magic way with animals, just as the psychic predicted, so we filled our house with animals: three dogs, two cats, a bird and a hamster.

He was starting to trip more often, so we had to watch him closely now. He held onto windows and door handles when he walked, and dragged his hands along walls to steady himself. Occasionally his legs would just give way, and he would suddenly fall to the floor. We would pick him up, brush him off and kiss his bruises away. Shortly after, we installed carpets in every room.

THE HILL

One day, his school was doing a Terry Fox Run, and all the kids were going to walk around the outside grounds of the school. Tristan proudly came home with his pledge sheet and announced he would do the walk. The next day, we went to his school and he set out with the rest of the kids. He was much slower and he tripped several times, but the teachers picked him up and he continued on.

On one part of the route, there was a small hill, and when Tristan reached the bottom of it, he stopped for a moment. I held my breath and waited for a cue. Tristan was fiercely independent, and we had learned to never help him unless he asked. The parents all turned to look at me, but I kept my eyes on Tristan. Then, we all watched as he fell to his knees, and began climbing up the hill on all fours. When he reached the top, a teacher scooped him up onto his feet, and he continued on his way. There wasn't a dry eye on the playground that day.

HEALTH FOOD STORE

With Tristan now settled in his new school, I took my resume and headed into town. My body was still very fragile, so I knew I needed to find a stress-free job. I applied at the local health food store, and met with the manager. She asked me if I had any experience in herbs and homeopathy. I told her I didn't have formal training, but that I used them myself for years. She was still unsure, but when I told her I knew about sports supplements, she hired me on the spot.

It had been several years since I had worked, and I was thankful to have something other than Tristan's illness to focus on. I loved the feeling of working again, and the store's atmosphere was very soothing. I could feel my body starting to unwind. I spent most of my time reading from the store library everything I could find about alternative therapies, energy and mysticism.

READING MY EYES

One day, we had an iridologist in the store doing readings for our clients. Iridologists believe that the eyes are like a body map and that all of our body parts are connected to a part of the iris, and that you can see the start of a disease before you feel any symptoms because the delicate eye fibres shift in colour, thickness and tone as the body's tissues change. My naturally curious nature got the best of me, and I signed up for a session.

She took pictures of my eyes with her high-powered medical camera and put them up on a large screen. She pinpointed all the pain spots in my body with incredible accuracy, and she pinpointed my digestive problems also. The flecks in my eyes mapped out certain organs that were showing signs of stress, and my body was also overly acidic. Then she pointed to a white circle along the outer edge of my iris. "You had a major shock in your life, an emotional shock that hit you hard about three years ago."

I nodded in disbelief. Tristan was diagnosed three years ago. It seems the shock of that day was forever etched in my eyes.

Today, if I look real hard, I can still see the ring's murky outline, faded in time now, as I continue to heal. It acts as a constant reminder of the undeniable connection between my emotions and my physical body.

MY MEDITATION

I had hoped that in time, Tristan's father would want to move closer to him and be more involved in his upbringing, but his dad remained living a distance away. I had always thought Tristan would have both parents involved in his day-to-day life, and with his dad's involvement, it would mean a much-needed break for my partner and me, and a chance for me to de-stress and tend to my health issues.

I confided in my spiritual intuitive, Cheryl, and she suggested I create a morning meditation around what I wanted. Meditation had become an important part of my healing, and I spent time in meditation every morning. Now, I would start my morning meditation with a new focus, so I began each morning with the following affirmation:

I wish to have Tristan's dad fully involved in his upbringing, so Tristan can have both parents involved in his life, while giving us the respite and support we need.

I meditated on this every morning, then I let it go. I hoped the Universe would sort out the rest.

THE LETTER (September 2003)

As time went on, nothing changed, and I began to feel angry that Tristan's father was still living so far away. I wrote him a letter asking that he move close to us and share equally in the care of our son, whose needs would only increase with time. I also outlined how hard Tristan's declining health had been on my health, and how I needed his support.

I had hoped his father would agree to equal parenting, but instead he demanded full custody of our son. I said no. He was newly married to a woman Tristan barely knew, and they lived in a ski resort, which would severely limit Tristan's mobility. We had reached a stalemate.

SHERIFF AT THE DOOR

Two months later, there was a knock at the door. A sheriff handed me an envelope. "Sorry," he said, "but this is for you."

It was a summons from my ex-husband. He was suing me for custody of our son. It was December 30th, our son's 8th birthday.

We were headed to court, and his lawyer was using my letter to my ex as evidence that I was unstable. Now I had to prove that I was mentally stable and capable of raising our son. I was furious.

I was ordered to see a counsellor who would assess my mental health and report back to the court. "It's not about the truth," explained our lawyer, "it's all about perspective. We have to prove to them that you're a capable, functioning mother. We can't show them any weakness."

I thought back to my meditation and wondered where it had all gone wrong. This is definitely not what I asked for. Or was it?

Over the next few months, we gathered all our resources and prepared our case. We finally had a date for mediation.

"Good news," said our lawyer. "We have a female judge who has spent the last 10 years taking care of her ailing husband. She'll be sensitive to your case."

I smiled. Maybe the Universe was at work here after all.

During court, my ex and I told our individual sides of the story. At the end, the judge's summary was clear: "You have a child that needs the help and support of both parents. You both need respite, and that includes your ex wife."

Shortly after, Tristan's dad moved to town, and we began to raise our son with equal time and equal respite for both.

The Universe *had* heard my prayers after all. But I would need its help even more in the upcoming months.

THE WHEELCHAIR (Fall 2004)

After the court case, we settled back into life as best we could, but with our legal bills, my on-going health issues and Tristan's continual decline, our relationship was feeling shaky.

Tristan was getting weaker fast, and he was tripping more often, so he became fearful of walking. We knew it was time to take the next step, the one we had all dreaded for years – it was time to get a wheelchair.

When his manual chair arrived, we sat it in the corner of his bedroom. We wanted him to get used to seeing it, then perhaps the reality of our situation could somehow be easier to accept. It was not.

Looking at that chair, with its big, shiny wheels and thick, black padding, chased away any last hold out for a cure or a change. There was no hope, and no turning back. *This is our new reality*, I thought. *It's finally here.*

"It's just there if you need a rest, Honey, and we can push you around in it for a bit," I explained to Tristan. I felt like a liar.

CHRONIC PAIN

I was still working at the health food store, and I continued to read and learn about alternative approaches to health and healing. I found comfort in alternative views of healing and disease, and while I had abandoned any hope of finding a cure for Tristan, I was hoping to find clues to my own health struggles.

The pain in my body had intensified, in particular, in my back, neck and shoulders, and there was never a moment when I wasn't in pain. I tried everything to relieve it – Reiki, chiropractor, massage, acupuncture and a host of lotions and potions. They all worked for awhile, but the pain would always return, and with more vengeance. I was fighting a formidable beast.

Medical intuitive Carolyn Myss says that all back pain stems from feeling unsupported. This certainly rang true for me. I felt angry at a Universe that would allow such a disease to take hold in my son's body. I had no family support, and no one to talk to who could really relate to what we were going through. I felt very, very alone.

PERIPHERALS

Our life was consumed with trying to get all the physical supports in place for Tristan. Up until this point we had been lifting and carrying him everywhere, but as time went on, it was becoming more difficult. It was now time to inquire about a wheel-chair accessible van and a ramp. We needed overhead lifts, showering and toilet aids and a new bed. We struggled to understand the different agencies to approach, and how the system worked. There was no parent pocketbook to refer to.

We were now on a steady round of doctors' visits as Tristan needed to go for regular heart and lung function tests and spinal x-rays. He now had a full-time health therapist and they created a team at school to provide in-classroom support and on-going skill assessments.

"Given his diagnosis, he's a shoe-in for support now," said one teacher's aide. "You won't have any problem getting any support for him now, especially with *that* diagnosis."

Tristan was struggling more and more with everyday tasks. He could no longer go to the bathroom or bathe himself, and it was becoming more difficult for him to feed himself. He couldn't open doors or drawers anymore, and he couldn't bend down to pick up anything because he couldn't straighten up on his own.

Now, I couldn't be more than a few feet from him because there was always something he needed, like a pencil that had rolled out of his reach or he couldn't stretch far enough to grab something. He was getting frustrated, and he often asked why little things that he could do before were now hard for him. I pretended I didn't hear him. I didn't know what to say.

THE NEUROLOGIST

It had come time to make a decision on whether Tristan would take steroids or not. Steroids are one of the only real treatment options for DMD, but the consequences can far outweigh the benefits, and their use remains a much-debated topic. Steroids promote greater strength, but they can cause damage to internal organs and cause emotional disturbances. Thankfully, Tristan's two families all agreed on a no-steroid approach, as we felt that quality of life was more important than anything else, so we declined. "It's not about *how long* you live," I would often say to Tristan, "it's about *how well* you live."

Tristan's neurologist made her distaste for our decision known at his next appointment. With Tristan still in the room, she turned to me and asked, "Does he realize that if he doesn't take steroids he won't live as long?"

Tristan turned and looked at me.

"Yes," I said, "we've discussed it as a family. We choose not to do steroids."

She scowled and left the room.

It would be many years later when I would be reminded of our family's philosophy. Tristan and I went to buy a kitten for our household, and we told the clerk that we were looking for an indoor/outdoor cat.

She refused to sell us one because she said outdoor cats don't live as long.

"It's not about how long you live," Tristan said to the clerk. "Cats are supposed to go outside. If he doesn't live as long, at least he had a good life."

Out of the mouth of babes....

THE HOME VISIT

That fall, two people from the health authority came to our house. A family member had called them because they were worried about my mental state.

"We just want to ask you a few questions," they said to me. We sat down on the couch and they started asking me questions from the list in their hands: *Did I know what day it was? Did I know what year it was? What was my middle name* and *Do I remember where I was born?*

I was furious at their insinuations. I refused to answer their questions. I listed all the stress we had been under for the past few years: three miscarriages, our move across the country and back, Tristan's diagnosis, the court case, our financial struggles and my health issues.

"I'm not crazy, I'm just really, really sad," I snapped. Then I asked, "Do either of you have a sick child?"

They both shook their heads no.

"Well, *if* and *when* you do, *then* you can come to me and tell me what to do. Until then, leave me alone."

I showed them the door. l never heard from them again.

THE ROCKING CHAIR

When they left, I sat in my rocking chair, the same chair I rocked Tristan in as a baby, and I started to cry. My partner came into the room and wrapped his arms around me.

"It's going to be ok," he whispered. "Everything that you're going through is for a reason, and you'll be able to teach it to other women."

I cried some more. How was I going to help anyone else if I couldn't even help myself? But somehow, his words made me feel a little bit better. Perhaps there was a purpose to this after all. I wish I knew.

TRIP TO EUROPE (summer 2004)

When Tristan was nine years old, his dad decided to take him to Europe. His father wanted to travel with him before Tristan lost the ability to walk all together. They were gone for six weeks and visited nine countries. Because of that trip, Tristan has a greater appreciation of the world and its many people and cultures, and I enjoy hearing him talk about his once-in-a-lifetime trip. I will forever be grateful for his dad's decision to take our son traveling.

This trip to Europe helped fill in a piece of the puzzle for me – when Tristan was gone, the pain in my body quickly stopped. I never realised just how much I had become accustomed to the pain. I had been living with chronic pain ever since Tristan's diagnosis, and its sudden departure was liberating! I had forgotten what feeling good felt like! I could clearly see the strong link between my physical and my mental state.

MY CRYSTAL BALL

That winter, I signed up for another course with Cheryl, the spiritual intuitive. I wanted to further delve into energy work and experience all it had to offer. I traveled to her beautiful home in the Interior every month for four months.

Cheryl taught us how to feel energy, and how to access other planes of consciousness. We did night travel and intense dream work and we spent hours in meditation. We learned how to use tarot cards, how to read auras, how to see chakras and how to channel. We learned how to work with Universal Laws, and how to use the Law of Attraction to manifest what we wanted in our lives.

During those sessions, I came to see Tristan's disease from a metaphysical place, and separate from the physical world. "Sometimes a loved one takes on a disease as a way to teach us important lessons that we wouldn't have learned otherwise," explained Cheryl. "It's their gift to us."

She continued, "When things shifted, you shattered. You were too rigid. The image I keep getting is truly of a crystal ball falling to the ground and shattering into a thousand pieces."

I understood. I was like the mighty Oak tree, strong and unbreakable, which I had prided myself on my whole life, but now, I needed to learn a different way. "You need to bend like the Willow," she said.

"This is your journey," she added. "*Stop making it wrong.*"

OUR WEDDING (Spring 2006)

The following spring, my partner and I got married. We chose a May wedding, because it was the same month that Tristan was diagnosed in. Tristan was getting weaker fast, and we wanted to have the wedding while Tristan was still walking. He and my future husband had matching tuxedos made, and seeing them, I marvelled at how handsome they were. I wished I could freeze-frame that moment in time forever.

We had a small outdoor wedding by the ocean. I toasted my husband and thanked him for all his love and support. I pulled out my journal, the one from seven years ago that I sat and wrote in, at my campfire, outlining all the qualities I wanted in a man. I read each one

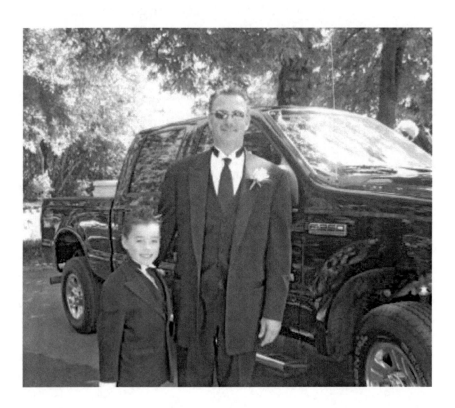

out loud – he had every single one of the traits on my list. Everyone could see the Universe *had* heard my prayers.

That fall, Tristan went into a wheelchair.

TWO WORLDS

For the next few years, we lived between worlds – the able-bodied and the disabled – but we didn't feel like we really belonged in either one. We felt unsure most of the time, but it was our new reality.

We struggled to create a new normal with Tristan's now full-time dependency on his chair. Looking back, I think he was thankful to finally be in a chair full-time, because at least he knew he would never trip and fall again, a kind of insurance policy against future hurts. But for me, the hurt continued in a different way, as I cried endlessly for the care-free runabout little boy that once was.

After nearly eight years of living through it all, we were bone-weary, and for the first time in my life, I was unsure of my own strength any-more. All our dreams were evaporating. All our best efforts seemed fruitless. No matter how much I bargained or cried, or screamed or prayed, no matter how many healers we visited, I could not change my son's path. My faith – my endurance – was crumbling.

My handsome men getting ready for our wedding. Tristan was having trouble walking and we knew soon he would no longer be able to walk, so we planned an earlier spring wedding. That fall, he went into a wheelchair full time.

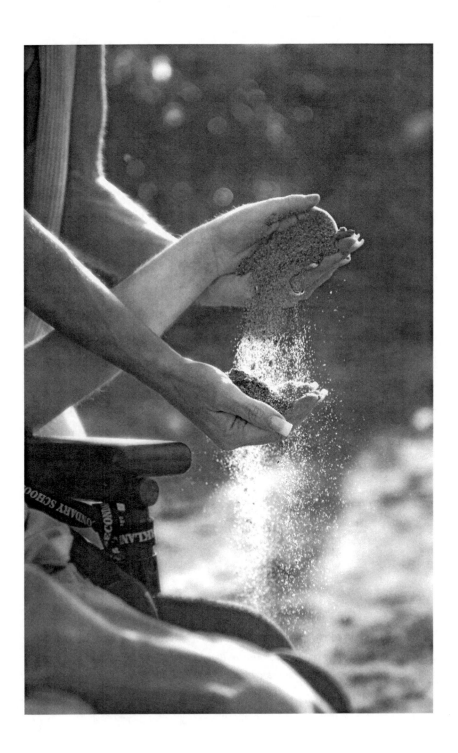

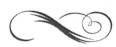

FIVE

Letting Go:
The Turnaround (2008 – present)

FOOT SURGERY, JUNE 2008 (7 years after diagnosis)

It's been five weeks since Tristan's foot surgery and I'm exhausted beyond words. The doctors slit his Achilles heel chords because the disease was causing his feet to curl up and inward, which set up its own chain of reaction that was causing his hips and spine to slowly move out of alignment.

It seems like a bitter joke to cut the heel chords of a child who can no longer walk. It's one of the many surgeries children with DMD go through as a matter of course, yet I often wonder if anyone really questions such practices, or if we just do them in an effort to feel like we are doing something.

Throughout the night, Tristan cries out in pain, and we turn him every half hour or so. I've moved into the back bedroom to be closer. My husband doesn't like it. The space between us is growing.

I sometimes watch other families as they go about their normal business and I remember what that used to feel like. I remember the little things... going to the playground, kicking around a ball, or just walking to the local store. The simple joys and rights of boyhood (and motherhood) are gone. The little milestones are replaced with big worries, and spontaneity and the feeling of joy have all but dried up.

He has called out in his sleep again, and again I make my way through the darkness to reposition him and try to make him comfortable again. I wrap my hands around his thick casts, holding there, for a moment, hoping my healing energy can somehow penetrate these thick clay and mortar encasings of his. I envision his tendons, red and throbbing, and the long incisions running up his leg. I am thankful he is medicated.

I look at his feet, now straight and true, with the proper 90-degree angle. They look 'normal' in their new positioning, and hopefully he can wear shoes again, something else he had to give up years ago because no shoes could sit on his tiny, contorted feet.

We are at yet another crossroads in this life-long journey of ours, and we must work to create yet another 'new normal' in this sea of constant change.

In rock climbing, there is a move called the faith hold: when the next rock is just outside a climber's reach, he must let go of his grip on one rock as he jumps for the other. For a moment he is suspended in air with nothing to hold on to. It's the ultimate act of letting go, but he must do it if he wants to continue the climb.

As I was pushed toward my own edge, I was desperate to find *my* faith hold. After living in the dark shadow of my son's diagnosis, I needed someone, *something* to grab on to.

After eight long years, I was about to reach that place, my turnaround, my salvation. Here I was about to learn the greatest lesson of all – the gift of surrender.

CASTS (Summer 2008)

After Tristan's foot surgery, he needed 24-hour care. He was heavily medicated and he was anxious about the pain. Our days and nights had become one big blur. We had to reposition Tristan's legs every hour, adding more pillows or taking some away to try to relieve the pressure on his heels. After eight weeks, the heavy casts finally came off, and his heels were bloodied and scabbed from the rubbing.

There were two long scars running from his heel into his lower calves, and his feet were pink and swollen. His feet, once contorted and curved up, now lay flat. *How ironic*, I thought, *perfectly straight feet, and they'll never be used for walking again.*

GARAGE SALE

That fall, we held a garage sale and piled all of Tristan's stuff together, things he hadn't been able to use for years but which I stubbornly held onto in hope, but there was no miracle coming.

So we piled his skateboard, his toboggan and his bike into a big box and took it outside to the driveway. A passer-by spotted his tiny lime-green bike with its $10 sticker and approached my husband.

"I'll give you 5 bucks for it," said the man. My husband was visibly annoyed.

"This isn't Mexico, there's no bartering here," my husband snapped. "The price is 10 bucks."

The buyer shuffled about and tried to negotiate some more. "Get the hell out of here," my husband barked.

The man left with a bag of nails and a puzzled look on his face. He would never know the real reason behind my husband's outburst. To this stranger, it was merely a bike for sale.

DRIFTING APART

During this time, my husband and I had drifted dangerously apart. We were like two strangers living under the same roof. In our sheer exhaustion and our fight to keep our heads above water, even the basic niceties and social graces had vanished between us. We passed each other in the hallway with barely a glance.

As Tristan's disease progressed, our lives continued to change. We used to love to visit the ocean, but now his chair could not make it through the heavy sand, so Tristan would sit off in the distance and watch us from afar. Eventually we stopped going altogether.

Our bedtime ritual was different now also. In the past, when Tristan felt scared or lonely, he would tip-toe down the hall and climb up into bed beside me. Now, he had to call for us and my husband would go get him and lift him into bed beside me. Eventually he stopped calling.

SECRET EMAILS

Tristan needed more care, but I was insistent on doing it myself. After all, I was his mother and Mother knows best, right? That's what good mothers do, they sacrifice for their children, or so I was taught, but the more I did, the more exhausted and angry I became, and the less my husband wanted to be around me. He spent more time away from home, and I was angry at his sudden absence.

After one particularly hard night, we had a fight and my husband left the house. I sat down and thought about the last few years. Our entire relationship had become one fight after another, and we were exhausted by it all. Caring for Tristan while trying to keep our marriage afloat had become nearly impossible. Where had we gone?

As I sat there, waiting for my husband to return, I opened up his laptop and clicked on the email icon. I opened up his messages and began to read. I didn't know what I was looking for, but I was looking for something, *anything* to feel connected to him again. There were dozens of work-related emails, and a host of emails from a woman with odd subject lines: hi again, see you soon and call me....

I sat for a moment and stared at the screen. The house was dead silent. *Should I open them?* I thought. Was this something I really wanted to know? Was this something I would be able to deal with, given all we were going through? Did I really want to go down this road? Did I want to open this Pandora's Box?

It would have been so easy to just close the computer and return to my life as if nothing had happened. Isn't that what my mother had done years ago? She had chosen to ignore the signs of my father's infidelity and remain on the safe, familiar road, then years later she suffered for it terribly. I didn't want that to happen to me. I needed to know.

I clicked on the first email and read it. Then I opened the next one, then the next. One by one I opened them all. I didn't stop until I read all the emails.

My heart sank. I felt the bitter sting of betrayal that my mother must have felt over 35 years ago when she finally found out about my father's other woman. I had stepped smack into my mother's footsteps.

After awhile, I heard my husband drive up. I ran out to meet him in the driveway. *Who was she?* I demanded to know. *What does she mean to you? How did you meet her? How long had it been going on?* He met her several months ago through work. She was a confidante, someone he could talk to about Tristan.

I fell to the ground, curled up into a ball and cried. *How could it have gotten to this point?* My head was filled with questions. *How were we going to get through this? Would he leave me? Should I confront her? Should I file for divorce?*

That summer was a blur as I tried to come to terms with it all. I pulled away from all friends and social gatherings, and I confided in no one. I sat by the ocean, I wrote and I cried, but some decisions had to be made. We needed a resolution.

We worked hard to keep our issues away from Tristan, and looking after him gave me something, anything to focus on rather than this new mountain sitting squarely in front of us.

THE LAWYER

I went to see a lawyer. I was going to file for divorce. After we went through all the required paperwork, he turned to me and said, "Do yourselves a favour. You and your husband need time away from your son. Go out to dinner. Let your husband know how important he is to you. This isn't about the other woman, it's about him not feeling needed."

I understood what he was trying to say: in the cloud of my son's illness, I had lost *us*. I had put my son first, and my husband a very distant second. At first, I defended myself, "That's what any mother would do - put her child before anything else...."

The lawyer shook his head. I had to face the truth. I was crippling my marriage. I had pushed my husband further away.

THE COUNSELLOR

I went to see a counsellor and we took a hard look at my past. We examined my working model and decided it needed a serious update. I had never learned what a healthy relationship was because I had no healthy role models in my life. I was confused about what a healthy relationship looked like – but I couldn't possibly create a healthy marriage from an unhealthy model, so we had to go back to the beginning.

Then my counsellor offered me his golden nugget of advice, one that I still use today: "A successful relationship is not 50/50, or even 100/100," he said. "It's really in how you look at it. It's 100/0. It's 100% you, and 0% the other person."

I must have looked stunned because he continued.

"Your husband has his work to do, and you have yours. Tend to yourself. Let him be. You can't control him, you can only control *you*. Your only responsibility is to be the best *you* you can be. It's called self-care."

I understood: if *I* was healthy, *we* would be healthy too. That was my only job at this point in time.

OUR RE-MARRIAGE

I continued working with the counsellor all summer long. I knew there was a chance that my husband would leave, and I now knew that I needed to let him go. I wanted him to *want to stay* because he *wanted to*, not because he felt he *had* to. I told him that Tristan and I would be okay, whatever he decided. It was one of the hardest things I ever had to do.

They say that *if you let something go and it comes back to you, it was yours. If it doesn't, it never truly was.* I had to let go of our marriage to free up the possibility of it coming back in a new way. It was scary, but also strangely liberating, and I felt parts of myself returning to me. I started feeling hopeful.

That fall, I felt my husband emotionally return to me. I never asked any questions for fear that it would cause us to fall backwards. We needed to move forward. The past was the past. So we worked to put our relationship back together, and we were able to build a solid union, one with greater awareness and a greater appreciation for each other. I also learned to let my husband share in Tristan's care. In doing so I was letting him know that he truly was a trusted and valuable part of our life. We were creating something new, whole and healthy again.

MY RE-WIRING

An evening at the movies provided another important shift in my healing. We went to see an IMAX movie called *Wired to Win: Surviving the Tour de France* which uses computer-generated imagery to take viewers into the mind of a racer on the Tour de France. Pathways of pain, fear and motivation are shown moving through the brains circuits so the viewer can see how that experience affects the athlete's brain and body.

Watching that movie changed something in me. As a competitive athlete, I had once felt *like them*. I had once been that focused and disciplined, and I remembered feeling that same *inner grrr* inside me that these athletes must have been feeling, but which I had lost. But I could feel it returning again!

As the camera sped along those neuro-pathways, I felt like the camera was moving through *my* body. As each image hit the screen, I could feel my own muscles firing up. Something inside me was shifting back into place. I was that athlete again, and I felt a surge of adrenaline rush through my body. I felt plugged in again!

When I got up the next day, I grabbed my training journal and headed for the gym. It had been six long years since I stepped inside a gym. It was time.

MY RE-TRAINING

My first few training sessions were a struggle. I had lost so much strength, and my body shook as I lifted each weight. I didn't like what I saw in the mirror either. My arms and legs were soft and fleshy, and my tummy spilled over my waist band. And my butt was flat! I was determined to get it all back.

I went home and calculated everything I had eaten the last two days. I was eating 600 to 800 calories over my usual intake, and the pages were filled with dense, sugary foods like bread, crackers, cheese and chips. I was living on a carbohydrate rollercoaster.

I printed off a blank calendar and I began to mark off my training days and what I would train. I then printed off blank food journals to write down everything I was eating. I was back on track, but I had lost six years of my life. I was now 47 years old. *Had too much time gone by? Could I train without pain? Could I get back in shape?*

Week after week I returned to the gym with journal in hand. I wrote down my sets, reps and weights for each workout. I was incredibly sore, but I could feel my body getting tighter every day. It felt great! I was able to up the ante slowly, week after week.

It would be almost a full year before I was able to use the same weights I had used when I quit training, but I had been re-wired.

Day after day, I returned to the gym, and my body was getting stronger and more flexible every day. I thanked it for its patience, and for all the lessons it had taught me. My body was slowly coming back, but it would still be quite some time before it was fully healed.

SEEKERS

The following spring, I returned to my roots and I started teaching classes on weight training and nutrition. The more women I trained, the more I could see a real desire for something more, something bigger than just creating a strong and healthy body. They wanted to find a spiritual connection to others and to the natural world around them. I was surrounded by seekers.

I knew what I needed to do: I had to use my experience to help other women. I wanted to teach them about the intimate connection between the physical and the spiritual. The Universe had planted the seeds in me for a new kind of fitness business, and I needed to make it grow.

MY RETURN

Sometimes we find our salvation in the strangest of places. I found mine in secret emails and in a nifty little movie about bike racers.

Over the next year, my body started to unravel and for the first time, I was free of pain. I was back to training full time, and my muscles were responding well to the training. My back, neck and shoulders had totally let go, and I was no longer plagued with mysterious body symptoms. My digestion was strong again, and I was sleeping soundly. I felt grounded and balanced again. I felt *human*.

Tristan was growing into a kind, sensitive and thoughtful boy who had long ago learned to surrender to the inevitability of his situation, and was a reminder to us all to do the same. He was in the groove of living between two households – his dad's city apartment and our country home – and there was no interruption in his schooling or his growing social life. He had a strong support team around him now who was ready and able to provide whatever he needed in equipment, school support, therapy and personal hygiene.

Our marriage was getting stronger every day as my husband and I continued to learn and grow together in a healthy way. We learned how to better ask for what we needed, and we learned how vitally important it was to remember to be patient and understanding at those times when we felt overwhelmed with it all.

I had come full circle, and back to the person I once was – healthy, joyful, loving and open to all that life had to offer. Life was still hard, and we still struggled with Tristan's on-going challenges, but as a

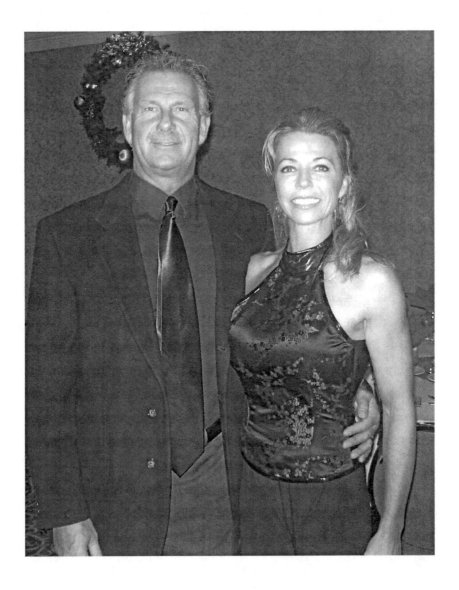

family we had gone to the centre of the storm and survived. We had endured. We now had new tools and new teachings to draw from, and we were better equipped. Our storm was finally passing.

After eight years, I came to understand that anger *and* peace, sadness *and* joy, fear *and* hope were all necessary and vital parts of the journey. I was walking through it now with open arms, and moving with our ebbs and flows. Here, in our vast ocean, there was no right or wrong, it just was, and we needed to walk it, to *feel* it and honour it, every step of the way. There was nothing for me to be afraid of anymore.

This is what my son's journey had taught me. This was our son's gift to us.

My dark night's journey was finally over.

Me and my hubby, Neil. We've weathered many storms throughout Tristan's journey, and are stronger than ever!

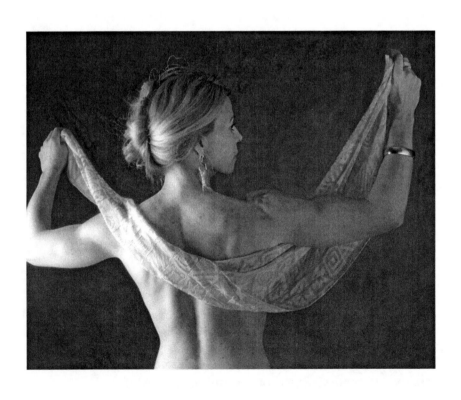

SIX

Loving What Is:
No Resistance

BACK SURGERY – LESSONS MY SON TAUGHT ME, JANUARY 28, 2011 (10 years after diagnosis)

On Friday, my son underwent an 11-hour back surgery to correct a severely crooked spine as a result of the wasting effects of muscular dystrophy.

The waiting part is always the worst. It is there, in the overwhelming silence of it all, where your mind starts to play tricks on you. Why isn't he out yet? They said he'd be out at 3 p.m… it's now 6 p.m…. did something go wrong? Why is everyone talking in hushed tones? What was that bell going off? Is my son okay?

Finally, around 5 p.m., we asked someone if they had an update. They told us to come back at 7 p.m. That was all they said. So family members dispersed, then returned several hours later. And we continued to wait.

The mind is a powerful thing, and left to its own devices, it can create all kinds of havoc. It did for me, sitting there, wondering if Tristan would be okay. Then I remember something a spiritual writer wrote many years ago that said the mind can only carry one thought at a time, and the best way to get rid of worry is to replace it another thought.

For me, I've always believed that the most powerful of all emotions is gratitude. So I mentally went through a whole list of things to be grateful for: the fact that the surgeon was one of the best in Canada, that my son was in one of the best facilities in Canada, that despite his chronic condition my son was otherwise healthy, with a strong, functioning immune system, and that if something terrible were to happen, he was in the right place at the right time.

I felt gratitude for other things: the fact that despite our past, his father and I could set aside our differences and sit together for hours in the same room, make conversation and stay focused on the task at hand. And our respective spouses did the same.

And I felt gratitude for my son, who, despite his daily challenges and progressive debilitation, pushes through each day, and amazes us with his inner resolve, his strength, and his sharp sense of humor. In that moment, I wiped away all my fear and sadness, and felt an incredible sense of safety and assurance that everything would be alright. In that moment, I sat with arms wide open, opening my heart to what is, and I felt grateful for being here, in this moment.

It's now Sunday evening and the rest of the family have returned to the Island, and I am alone, sitting beside my son in his hospital room. My son is sleeping and I am watching him sleep. I watch his tiny chest go up and down with every breath, and I am thankful for this. I run my hand up and down his tiny spine, and I feel the dozens of staples holding his long incision together. I feel the long tubes embedded deep into his lower back to help remove any signs of infection, and I watch the medicine bag slowly release its drippings into the tube in his tiny hand, and I am thankful to be a part of his continuing journey, wherever it may take us. However I have defined health, I trust that his body is capable of doing all it can do. And in this moment, that is enough.

This is how it's always been – Tristan and me, together as one. It's always been that way, he and I. And I pray it will continue that way for many years.

REFLECTIONS

Living through our son's journey has been our family's greatest blessing. The journey was long and the lessons were hard, to be sure, but I am thankful for every step.

We all must go through our own dark night if we are to live a full, rich life. It can be profoundly unsettling, and the desire to jump the cue is strong. Here, we are called on for a spiritual response, not a therapeutic one, and we must draw on our inner strength and faith to get us through.

Most people see suffering as negative. We're taught that we should move through the painful parts as quickly as possible, and we learn to dampen our pain through drugs, alcohol, working, shopping, eating, affairs and other outs. Don't. Don't stifle it. Don't rush the process.

Don't jump the cue. Suffering needs a voice. Give it one. Listen to it, or it will be forced to come out down the road, expressed as physical or mental pain, dysfunction or disease.

For me, my body was a barometer for everything in my life. What started out as a host of physical maladies one after another was my body expressing what my spirit couldn't – let go of the old, open up to the new, live with fresh eyes and an open heart. Now my body has become my trusted friend, one that always lets me know when I'm living in my truth or not. I continue to be amazed at its accuracy.

Traveling through your dark night is a lot like lifting weights. You can't rush the process if you want to see real results. You need to keep on the path, day after day, and to trust that changes are happening at a cellular level even when you can't see it. You have to dig deep and draw on your inner strength. You have to know when to push through and when to back off. Every step of the journey, like every rep in the gym, moves you toward greater health. It's about growing into your greatest potential, living with purpose and passion. It's about living your best life.

LIFE'S PURPOSE

After a long hiatus, I headed back to the gym. I had been awakened and I was clear on my purpose, and the old training model seemed outdated now, with its focus solely on building *physical* health. I knew I needed to create something unique, something that would resonate with women everywhere.

One year later, McCoy Fitness and Health was born. Its guiding philosophy was simple:

To live with passion, purpose and intent,
To live from the inside out,
To live with divine health,
To live as co-creators of our world.

Today, through on-line programs, weekend retreats, seminars, tele-conferences, and trade shows I have the privilege of working with women from all over the world.

THE BLISS™ PROGRAM

I hope you enjoyed reading *One Rep at a Time* and I trust you will thoroughly enjoy your **8-Week BLISS™ Body Makeover Program**. It is truly unlike any other program around. I couldn't have taught it any other way really, knowing what I know now. Please email me as you work through the program. I'd love to hear from you.

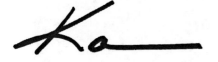

FINAL THOUGHTS – LEG DAY

Today is leg day, and I'm heading into the gym with training journal in hand. As I put on my gloves I bend down to open up my journal, and I glance at the front cover. At the top of the journal the word "INSPIRE" is printed on it. Inside, there is a little hand-written note from several women who gave me the journal as a gift. "You are an inspiration to us all, Karen. Thank you for all that you do."

I smile. It was what the psychic predicted years ago: *We're all here for a purpose, and your purpose is to inspire.*

Back then I couldn't hear it, given my health and where I was in my life. Now, looking down at those words scribbled there, I now understand that my life's purpose was always there waiting. I just had to step into it.

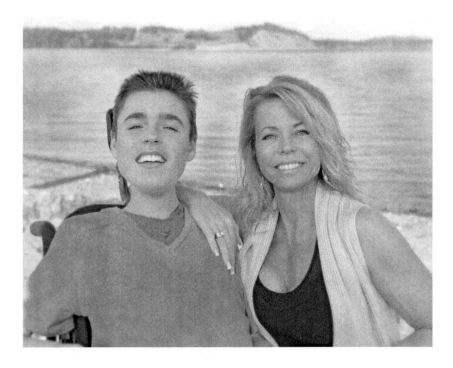

No resistance.

Years ago I measured success by how perfect my biceps were or whether I won or lost a show. I now know that our victories occur far away from stage lights and trophies. In my quiet spaces, I have been able to heal my spirit and my body, and I am thankful that my body was strong enough to endure what it did, and for as long as it did. But my greatest victory has been the chance to travel on this amazing journey with my son, and to continue traveling on it wherever it takes us.

Let go.

People ask me why, after 30 years, I continue to train as hard as I do. I list any number of reasons: to stay strong, to stay lean, to look good and to function well.

I lift for health reasons, it's true, but I also lift because I feel a connection to my power and to something beyond what I can see. I lift so I can tune into a Universe that's always talking to me, and trying to show me a better way. I lift because it reminds me that I'm still here.

I lift out of a deep respect for all things, seen and unseen.

I lift out of a respect for the human body in all its workings.

I lift for my son.

I lift because I can.

Arms wide open...

Me and Tristan at the ocean's edge, 2011. We are grateful for every moment of every day we get to spend on our journey together.

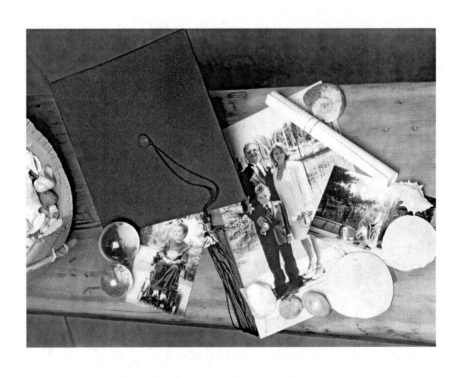

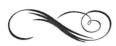

SEVEN

Graduation:
Milestones

GRADUATION DAY, JUNE 2010

On Monday, we went to our son's grade eight graduation.

While everyone clapped as each graduate accepted his or her certificate, I was sitting quietly in the back row, hiding my tears behind big sunglasses.

See, my son was never supposed to make it this far. When he was 10, he was diagnosed with a serious and degenerative form of muscular dystrophy that causes every muscle in his body to slowly deteriorate over time.

I can hear one doctor's voice like it was yesterday: "He'll be in a wheelchair by 10." (True). "His lungs and heart will weaken." (True). "He'll lose the use of his arms too." (True). "He'll be gone in his twenties...

In our family, we mark each milestone by taking little steps, because big steps are too far into the future and too uncertain.

Our next milestone is to watch him graduate from high school.

We've learned to not just live for today, but to live for the moment. There's joy and richness here, in the moment, and living in the moment, for any of us, is the only place where we have power.

Life is a continual dance of holding on and letting go. My son's body reflects that dance as it holds on and lets go, trying to hold on to what-

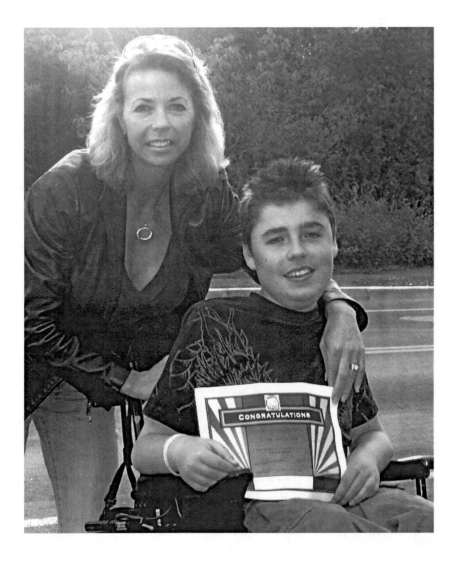

ever strength it can while letting go little by little into the inevitable. And I am there, beside him, helping him to move with that flow, as I move with my own flow. I am thankful for all his disease has taught me and I am thankful my son has included me in his life's journey.

Love your family. Be with them, really be with them. Muscle into every moment. Pay attention to your life. Accept what is, and be grateful, really grateful, for what you have. Say it out loud. Say it often.

Live with arms and heart wide open. Stay open to the possibilities. Lean into your sharp points, and know that you have the fortitude and strength to make it through your own dark night.

Some people think a graduation for grade eight is silly. Not for us. For us, it's another chance to be able to celebrate our son's life and all the gifts his journey has taught us.

We are thankful for having the chance to enjoy yet another milestone, and we have come to learn that life's greatest treasures are to be found deep within these milestones. And life is not to be endured, but it's to be lived with great courage and love and respect for all things seen and unseen. It's to be lived one step at a time. One Rep at a Time.

TODAY

Our family lives on beautiful Vancouver Island, close to the ocean and hidden among towering Douglas fir trees and the odd gnarly arbutus tree. Our house is always filled with animals, and currently

Me and Tristan at his Grade 8 Graduation ceremony, as he proudly displays his graduation certificate.

we have a dog and three cats and a growing pet cemetery out back. We are visited regularly by squirrels, eagles, barn owls and the odd raccoon that sometimes comes into the house late at night to eat out of the cats' food dish.

Tristan is now 16 years old and enjoying high school. He plans on going to university, but he has not yet decided what he wants to study. It lies somewhere between creating devices for disabled people or designing the next best sports car. His biggest disappointment is that he will never be able to drive a Ferrari. He is anxiously waiting for the day when he can live independently on his own.

Tristan's favourite subject is history, and he loves learning about

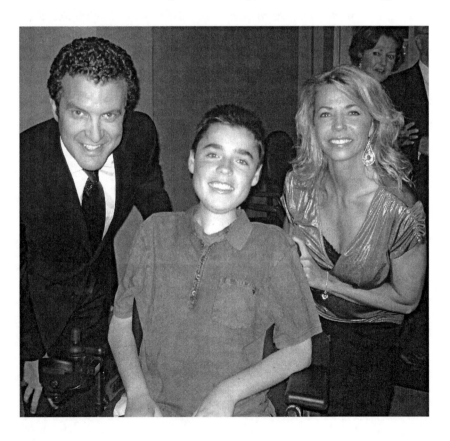

important historical times that changed the world. He also enjoys reading about my mother's upbringing through various emails, and he listens to his uncle's stories about travel and living through the Second World War. He enjoys watching programs on history and documentaries, and his favourite TV show is BBC's *Top Gear*, a show that includes cars, comedy and *middle aged men falling over*. He loves listening to jazz and rock, and his favourite rock bands include The Who, The Rolling Stones, Eric Clapton and Creedence Clearwater Revival.

Our son has traveled to 12 different countries, and his favourite is England. He hopes to one day live there part-time. He is drawn to Buddhism with its emphasis on peace and balance, and its affinity for the natural world. He gets frustrated when people only believe what they can see with their own eyes. He believes there is so much more which cannot be proven by science alone. He thinks people who are open to the possibilities of other beings and other worlds are much more interesting than people who value science alone.

Tristan's hope is that advances in stem cell research will bring forth a cure for MD and other diseases. He is well aware of all the implications of his disease and how it changes over time. He remembers walking, and feeling the grass under his feet. He remembers walking downhill and feeling the pressure in his legs when he did.

Tristan continues to teach everyone around him about tenacity

---

Meeting funny man Rick Mercer at Victoria Foundation's 75th Anniversary celebration at the Empress Hotel in Victoria, BC. Tristan is the Foundation's youngest donor, and the Tristan Graham Children's Foundation *raises money for the SPCA through our annual* Walk a Mile in Our Shoes *Walkathon.*

and patience, and he shows us all how to live with an open heart, and unafraid. He has come to accept his journey with incredible maturity and insight. When things get tough, he often says, "That's just the way it is, we can't do anything about it."

Our son's passion and empathy for animals has led us to create the **Tristan Graham Children's Foundation**, managed by **The Victoria Foundation**. Our five-kilometre fundraiser – *Walk a Mile in Our Shoes* – is held the third weekend in May. The goal is to raise awareness of all children living with Duchenne Muscular Dystrophy, and to help Tristan help his favourite things – animals. Every year we give to abused and abandoned animals in BC. It's our way of paying it forward. We are also donating one dollar from the sale of each book to go to his Foundation.

To date, Tristan is the Foundation's youngest donor and he is an example for all young adults to get involved at any age. For more information or to donate, please visit www.victoriafoundation.bc.ca

Our family has created a website www.tristangraham.com to support others going through similar challenges. Know that you are not alone. Please drop us an email. We'd love to hear from you.

Blessings,

Karen

&

TRISTAN

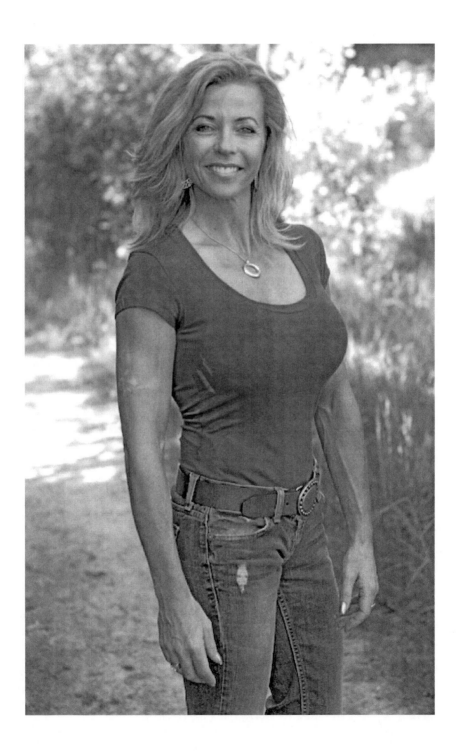

PART II

The 8-Week BLISS™ Body Makeover Program

Get lean, fit, shapely
and sexy for life!

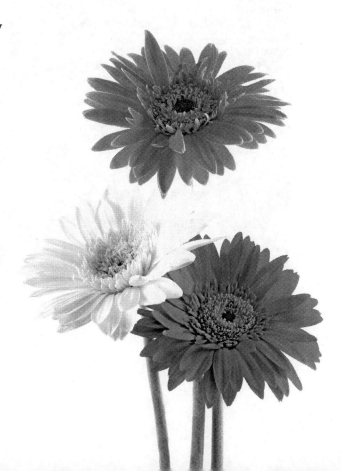

BLISS™ – BodyLife Integrated Sculpting System™

Physical Aspects

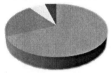

- Clean Nutrition
- Weight Training
- Cardio
- Supplements

Spiritual Aspects

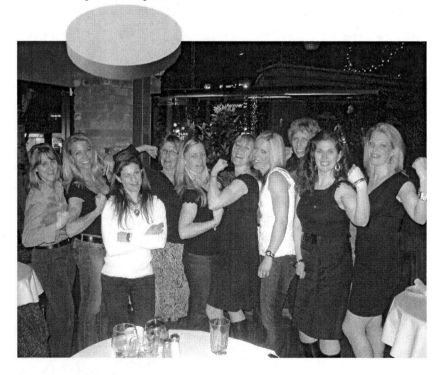

ONE

What is BLISS™ and How Does It All Work?

The BLISS™ Program (BodyLife Integrated Sculpting System™) is unlike any other training and lifestyle program. BLISS™ is a complete coaching program that uses the power of weight-training, cardio, clean nutrition and quality supplements to create a lean, healthy body, but it doesn't end there. For true health and wellness, we must harness the power of our mental, emotional and spiritual bodies to create a complete system of health, vitality, energy and wellness *on all levels*, for LIFE!

- TRAINING: The principals behind the 8-Week BLISS™ Body Makeover Program are based on the principals of body building. I prefer to call it *body sculpting*, because that eases women's

---

Celebrating the success of my first-ever on-line training program with 12 amazing women who did the program and who had amazing transformations! They're living proof that on-line training is a great way to train: affordable, practical and hugely successful! You rock, ladies!

minds a bit, but body building and body sculpting is the same thing. With BLISS™, you are the sculptor and weights are your tools. We'll look at debunking the myths around women and weights later.

- DIET: BLISS™ teaches you about science-based clean eating practices. So throw out your Canada Food Guide, turn off the Internet, and ignore the advice of others. I'll teach you the real deal about clean eating!
- CARDIO: How much cardio do we need? Not as much as you think. In our program, we use it *wisely.*
- SPIRITUAL: Notice how the spiritual aspect gets its own pie chart, because we have to include the spiritual and emotional in everything we do. It's about living, eating and training with eyes wide open.
- SEASONS: Our workouts change from season to season, and so does our eating. It's about living in tune with Mother Nature. That's the only way to build a strong immune system and optimum health and vitality!

HOW DOES IT ALL WORK?

It's quite simple really. Since you purchased this book, you now have access to my web site which holds the workout videos, cards, articles, packages… everything you need for the next 8 weeks! Here you'll find your **8-Week BLISS™ Body Makeover Program**.

1. Go to www.mccoyfitness.ca
2. Click on the tab **Karen's Book** on the left hand side. You'll then be directed to the **Workout Page**.

3. Access is with your BLISS™ password – blissbody

4. Voila! You're in the program. Everything you need is found here.

The program consists of **3 Phases** which you'll move through consecutively. Don't forget to download the **Training** and **Nutrition and Lifestyle Packages** found in each phase as these will be the peripherals you'll need to help you create your BLISS™ body!

PHASE ONE – WEEKS 1 AND 2
BUILDING A STRONG FOUNDATION!

- TRAINING: In Phase One, it's all about building a strong foundation. Your training will consist of two rotating whole body workouts – lower body and upper body – which are designed to strengthen ligaments and tendons, and to prepare the body for future overload. With this workout, you'll be training 3 days a week and you can do it at home or in a gym. These workouts will also fill in weak gaps and will improve any injuries and imbalances that could be contributing to poor posture or pain. We also look at cardio, plyometrics and stretching.

- BODY MEASUREMENTS: Your initial Body Measurement Sheet is here, and I strongly encourage you to follow along and take the required measurements, and take your 'before' photos. We'll be doing this again at the end of the eight weeks. You also have a **Tracking Sheet** to keep you on top of your training and eating. You can also enter to win the **Best BLISS™ Body Makeover Contest** that I run every month. You'll win lots of fun prizes and I'll feature you on my site!

- NUTRITION: We start to build your nutritional foundation with quality **macronutrients**, and we take the man-made, refined products out of our diet. You'll also learn why I call **protein** the magic bullet, and you'll learn to look at **carbohydrates** in a whole new light (they are not the enemy), and the role of healthy fats. We check out calories and the importance of writing them down.
- **Mind / Spirit:** We look at shifting your inner landscape and creating strong, workable **goals** and fresh **beliefs** that empower and uplift you! This is one of the key elements of my BLISS™ Program.

PHASE TWO – WEEKS 3 TO 5
STRENGTHENING THE HOUSE!

- TRAINING: For the next 3 weeks, we up the ante and head to the nearest gym where we increase your training intensity while upping our weights, which ramps up our metabolism while creating more shape and tone! We learn about the role of cardio and how less is actually more (that's right!). And we learn how to find our lifting weight in order to maximize our results.
- NUTRITION: We look at the importance of **eating in season,** and eating **close to the earth.** We learn about our **body's natural daily rhythms** and some tips and tidbits for honouring ourselves by living in sync with our natural rhythms. We touch on calories, and we learn that label reading is murky, and that not all calories are created equal.
- MIND / SPIRIT: In this phase, we look at **The Law of Allow-**

ing. It is one of my favourite Universal Laws to live by and it will transform your life and the lives of everyone around you in profound and uplifting ways!

PHASE THREE – WEEKS 6 TO 8
YOUR DEFINING MOMENT!

- TRAINING: Our final 3 weeks consist of breaking through our barriers and upping the ante again. We need to hit those lovely muscles of yours from different angles so we change up the exercises, reps and sets for ultimate shape and tone! This is truly your defining moment!

- BODY MEASUREMENTS: Send in your final Body Measurements sheet and your 'before' and 'after' photos and let's see how you did! Enter to win the **Best BLISS™ Body Contest!** See how you stack up! Loads of fun, and motivating too! More info on your Training web page.

- NUTRITION: By now, you've got your eating under control and you've lost some weight. Great! You're starting to see things taking shape, so now we want to keep that momentum going! I introduce my own food pyramid, called the **Clean Zone Pyramid** with some tips on how to use it in your everyday life. And I include my list of clean shopping labels that you can find in almost any traditional grocery store. I also offer tips on eating consciously and other tools to help you stay lean, healthy and energized.

- MIND / SPIRIT: We look at shifting our perspectives by questioning what kind of **glasses** we're wearing. Change your glasses, change your life! We also look at holding the reins to create incredible and lasting success. My final lesson has been my greatest tool for change, the **Arms Wide Open** philosophy of living. When we stay open to our journey, we can hear the whisperings of the Universe, and our bodies and spirits stay supple and strong.

TWO

Goals and YOU!

Did you know the number one reason for failure to get in great shape / lose body fat, etc. is the lack of clearly-defined, written goals? How many times have you said to yourself, "I want to lose weight, feel healthy, fit into my old clothes, look like I did when I was younger." Good goals, to be sure, but vague and without any *punch*!

I am firmly convinced that the most important part of getting in great shape is simply *making up your mind to do so.* You get in shape by setting goals and thinking about them *all day long.* If you don't channel your mental energies properly, even the best program won't help because you will always sabotage yourself.

What do you want to accomplish and in what time frame? Write your goals down in *present tense* (very important!) and be specific. Get rid of *I'll try* or *I can't.* That is defeatist language.

Example:

Rather than say...	*Say...*
I want to look great.	I am on my way to dropping 20 pounds by (date)!

I want to feel better.	I am on my way to slipping into size 4 jeans by (date)!
I want to have nicer arms.	I am already seeing my arms tighten more every day!

It's *your* turn! What do you want to accomplish at the end of the *8-Week BLISS™ Body Makeover Program*?

My training / eating / weight goal(s) to be completed at the end of 8 weeks include: ...

Think hard about what you want to see come into your life! Don't put limits on it... silence that inner critic for a minute! You'll have a chance to write these down in the section entitled Creating Your New Belief Map a little later. You can then transfer these statements to your FOCUS Cards found on the BLISS™ Workout Page.

Your **BLISS™ FOCUS Cards** are an important tool to create strong, workable and supportive goals that will help you navigate through the program and through your life. The cards will help to hardwire your desires into your brain so they will become a reality. Start with 3 or so goals at a time, then once you attain these, create fresh ones every 3 to 6 weeks! Life is always changing, and your goals will change as you grow. It's the nature of things.

Remember, as you read each goal, *feel it as if you already have it!* This part bears repeating because it's so important. *Walk as if.* Get all your five sense on board. Know that you are capable and worthy.

THREE

Flexing Our Physical,
Mental and Spiritual Muscles

FLEXING OUR PHYSICAL MUSCLES

My 8-Week BLISS™ Body Makeover Program will help carve and shape your physical body in new and exciting ways. The benefits of weight training may seem obvious, but let's go over them again. Some may surprise you!

- BOOST YOUR METABOLISM: Remember, your *metabolism is in your muscles*. Studies show that five pounds of added muscle helps you burn almost 200 extra calories a day – even at rest. In this way, your muscles are working for you 24/7.
- INCREASE YOUR ENERGY: If you feel too tired to train, then that's a sure clue that you have to train! Movement creates energy. Simple!
- CUT THE CRAVINGS: Weight training helps to level out blood sugar levels, resulting in fewer cravings and weight loss.
- STRENGTHEN BONES: Bone loss starts in your mid-thirties

with a decline in hormones, and activities like swimming and running are great, but they don't hit the bones in a way that causes them to strengthen and thicken. Training with weights has been shown to halt, and in some instances reverse, bone loss.

- STAND TALLER: Next time you're standing outside your gym, take a look at how women walk after leaving the gym. Not only are you strengthening all the postural muscles, you walk with more confidence and more energy in your stride.

- STAY FLEXIBLE: It's one of our greatest myths: weights make you inflexible. It's untrue – *not stretching* makes you inflexible. Any athlete will become inflexible if they don't stretch. Using a full range of motion in weight training keeps your joints flexible. I'll show you how.

- HAPPY, HEALTHY HORMONES: If you suffer from hormonal havoc, go train. It's amazing the difference it can make (I never experienced hormonal fluctuations until I *stopped* training!).

- IMPROVE YOUR BALANCE AND COORDINATION: As we age, we naturally lose our balance and coordination. When we start lifting weights, in particular free weights (not machines), the body is forced to become better coordinated in its efforts.

- ELIMINATE BACK PAIN: Proper training helps the back do its job properly, because its location in the body is the main pivot point for all work in the body from head to toe. But according to back specialist John Sarno, back pain has roots in the spiritual. He has found that muscles get 'locked' in a holding pattern of stress and anger. (This was certainly true in my journey). For more information, read John Sarno's *Healing Back Pain* or visit www.healingbackpain.com.

- HELPING YOUR BODY HOLD: A trained body has a much greater capacity to 'hold' a health practitioners' work (chiropractor, physiotherapist, acupuncturist, etc.) for longer periods of time. A toned muscle can hold its place more effectively.

FLEXING OUR MENTAL MUSCLES

With BLISS™, we also build and flex our mental muscles in new and exciting ways. Like any muscle, the more you use your mental muscles, the stronger they get, which translates into success in all areas of your life.

- CREATE A NEW LIFESTYLE: They say it takes 21 times to make a new habit stick. I think they've got it all wrong. Look at anyone who exercised for a few months, got great results, then you see them again and they let it go because 'life got busy' and now they can't find the time to get back to it. Why did this happen? Because it became a *habit*, but not a *lifestyle*.

  You can drop a habit but you can't drop a lifestyle. Brushing your teeth is a lifestyle, and you wouldn't think of dropping that. We need to think of exercise and eating in the same way. So let's look at creating a new *lifestyle*!

- BREAK THROUGH BARRIERS: Nothing feels better than accomplishing something you didn't think you could do! Seeing a woman lifting a 20-pound dumbbell for the first time, I smile because I know she is breaking through her own limiting beliefs about herself, and shedding female stereotypes.

In the BLISS™ Program, you will write down your weights, reps and sets, so you have a reference point to look back on. When you look back, you'll be amazed at how far you've come. What you thought was impossible, you now lift with ease. Feeling proud of yourself is one of the greatest gifts we can give to ourselves.

- RENEW YOUR HEALTH VOWS: Many people think that once you learn how to exercise and eat well, it becomes second nature. Well, yes and no. Sure, the more you do something, the more likely you will stick with it, but we all know that's not always the case. I can't begin to tell you the number of women who have said they trained for a period of time, sometimes for several years and then they quit, for reasons they often don't understand.

  With BLISS™, you'll renew your vows to yourself every day with your BLISS™ FOCUS CARDS. Once you learn this valuable lifestyle tool, staying on track with your eating and training becomes easier.

- FALLING OFF THE BANDWAGON: How can falling off the healthy eating or training bandwagon be good for you mentally? When you fall off, *you have to get back on*, which takes willpower, and you build trust in yourself. Life is not about staying on your game all the time. I've literally fallen off thousands of times, but I just get back up. There will always be situations that will cause us to lose our grip – weddings, holidays, vacations. Consider these practice runs in building your 'bandwagon strength'. As the song goes, "Pick yourself up, dust yourself off, start all over again!"

- DELAY GRATIFICATION: One of my favourite books is *The Road Less Travelled* by Scott Peck. In this amazing book, he teaches that responsible, mature adults learn to delay gratification. In other words, you do the tougher stuff first, and then you can enjoy the rest. A classic example is children learning to eat their meat and veggies before diving into dessert. It's the same with training – if you leave it until the end of the day, you may not do it. Try to do it earlier in the day, before you run out of time! Say yes to your training before you indulge in other things. Create that mental promise to yourself.

FLEXING OUR SPIRITUAL MUSCLES

BLISS™ helps you connect to primal power and inner strength as you access that amazing world of possibilities behind the veil. By now you know that life is lived both in front of and behind your eyes.

- MY ZEN: When I walk into a gym, my focus shifts. As I approach a weight, my mind empties, my breathing slows and I go quiet. I don't hear or see anyone and the rhythm takes me away to some other place. I become one with the weights. Science has called it many things – the flow, a walking meditation, the mind muscle connection. I just call it my *Zen*.

    Most women miss this most amazing part of weight training because most trainers don't know how to teach it. This is a huge loss to clients (and trainers) everywhere. For my clients, lifting is as much a spiritual practice as it is a physical one. Lifting helps access our physical power, yes, but it also helps us to access and grow in spirit. When we are expanding, we are in a state of optimal, *divine* health. This is an important part of BLISS™ – flexing and building our spiritual muscles.

- STRENGTHENING OUR CHAKRAS: When we lift, we are connecting to that deepest, most primal part of us, our inner power and our spirit. This can be further explained by viewing the body's chakra system.

   Within the body is a chakra system. Each area of the body corresponds to an energy vortex. There are seven of these energetic powerhouses in total. Of particular importance in weight training are the first three chakras from pelvis to solar plexus. When I started training, I felt like I was walking *from my pelvis*, as if my pelvis was leading the way. At the time, I knew nothing

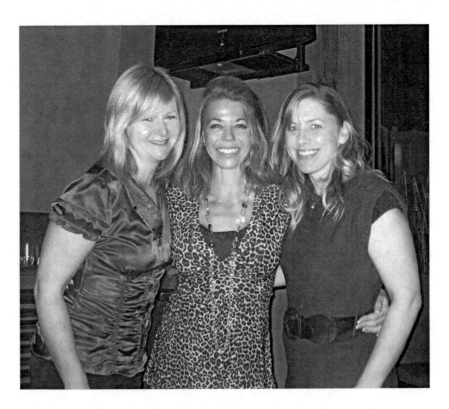

about chakras, but when I learned about energy, I understood: I had activated my power (third) chakra. I could even 'see' a golden-orange light emanating from there.

I see this in women who weight train all the time. They seem to lead from their pelvis, their power place, and you can almost feel the power ooze from their energy field. (Note: a full discussion of the charka system is beyond the scope of this book, but I highly recommend you become acquainted with this energetic system for optimum health and vitality.)

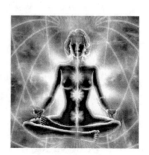

- VISUALIZING SUCCESS: During my first contest, I was unknowingly using the power of visualization while rehearsing my routine over and over again in my head. I learned that the key is to use all your senses and to actually feel like it's happening in real time. This is a key factor in successful visualization and in my BLISS™ Training program, and once learned, it's a pathway to creating great successes in your training and your life!

When you train, envision how you want to look *and feel* (put some Zen into it), and you will start seeing shifts happening. Your body won't change overnight, but it *will* change. It takes

I just love these gals – both started out as my clients and they trained under me for two years. They loved the life so much they both became trainers! Welcome to the team, ladies! (Michelle Bourgeois, left, and Angela Turnbull, right).

time to shift and mould muscle and tissue, but with consistent work and strong visualization, it *will* happen.

- WOMEN AND POWER: This book follows my journey through gaining and losing power and its effect on my health. Our power is the most precious thing we have, and it is the portal to creating true health and wellness. Sadly, society is not the only vehicle which can cause us to lose power: women often do it to themselves too. Women have historically minimized themselves out of fear of challenging the status quo, challenging current relationships, or fear of their own power.

Our bodies can be our greatest strength and also our greatest fear. A strong female body epitomizes power and sensuality, but it's a double-edged sword. Being too strong can be a threat to others. We secretly want to feel powerful and strong, yet, we short-change ourselves to appease others (and ourselves). And so we live on this see-saw of *I want this but I'm afraid of what it will look like to others.*

I often see this dichotomy at work when women first meet me. "I don't need to look like you, I just want to be healthy," they often say. But what they're really saying is they're afraid of wanting to look good and/or they feel they either don't deserve it or that it's unattainable. They lower their standards so they're not disappointed. They end up shooting for the moon (kind of) when they could be shooting for the stars. How do we manoeuvre in a world where we continually run the risk of alienating men, other women, family, and community if we grow? Marianne Williamson's *Return to Love* says it all:

"Our deepest fear is not that we are inadequate. Our deepest fear is that we are powerful beyond measure. It is our light, not our darkness that most frightens us. ... Your playing small does not serve the world. There's nothing enlightened about shrinking so that other people won't feel insecure around you."

Our getting healthy acts like a mirror that highlights other people's lack of success. The best thing any of us can do is *live by example*. We need to light our own fire and ignite our own spirit and live the life we are meant to live. Women are the most powerful force in the Universe. We deserve to celebrate this.

FOUR

Beliefs and YOU – What Do YOU Believe?

As a trainer, a big part of my work is building the body's muscu-lature. But in my experience, the most often overlooked muscle which *truly* defines whether we are successful or not is **our BRAIN!**

I'll say it again: *health and wellness is an inside job*, because long before we're sidelined with injury, or a tree falls on our car and we can't get to the gym, or we're abducted by aliens, we end up giving up our goals. Why? Because when it comes to successful training and eating habits, our underlying beliefs determine our success.

To make lasting change, we need to do some digging. This is un-comfortable work, but if I'm going to help a client be all she can be

---

A summer solstice celebration with another group of on-line training clients who lost a total of 163 pounds over a 10-week period! Looking awesome, ladies! I had women from as far away as Japan, Saudi Arabia and Florida train with us. Unfortunately they couldn't make the dinner!

in body, mind and spirit, accessing the deeper recesses and throwing light on her belief system is absolutely necessary for her success.

More often than not, I'm met with resistance, so I gently push through. How far I can go is dependent on how willing my client is. In other words, how much pain is she in now and how willing is she to take pain on will determine her success. *The only way out is through.* We need to update our Belief Maps and state strong, clear goals to get us there!

BELIEFS VERSUS VALUES

One of the biggest roadblocks I see is the fear of letting go of our beliefs because we often define ourselves by our beliefs, and we feel we

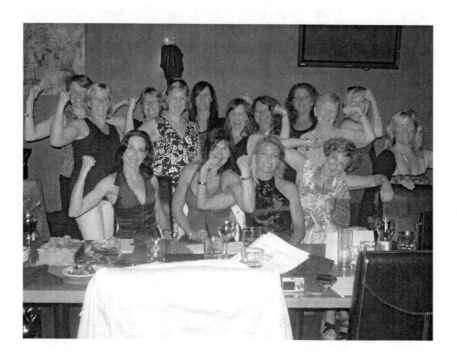

can't live without them. But that's because we often confuse beliefs for values, but they are different.

- BELIEFS ARE SUBCONSCIOUS. Like an iceberg, you may not even understand that they're running your life. Buried deep in the oceans of your mind, you have set patterns and beliefs about food, love, relationships, exercise and more. The successful person questions them all the time, to see if they 'hold water'.

- VALUES ARE CHARACTER TRAITS THAT WE CARRY FOR LIFE. They are our personal code of conduct – integrity, helpfulness, honesty, charity and being forthright. Living in agreement with one's values is fulfilling and life-affirming. Values, like character, do not change. Values are linked to your purpose in life and they do not change.

So many people don't want to let go of their beliefs but when I ask them why they believe a particular thing, they often say, "That's what I was taught to believe." We've adopted beliefs, without question. As we age, we're supposed to allow our beliefs to change. That's what responsible adults do (we used to believe in the tooth fairy, remember?). If we don't, we're cutting off our growth and we're running from ego rather than from our true authentic self.

Beliefs can seem so solid and unchangeable, more like facts, but they are clearly a choice, and once we learn this, we can learn that it's okay to let go of beliefs that no longer serve us.

BELIEF VERSUS WILLPOWER – NO CONTEST

Do you feel like you just don't have the willpower to stick with your new healthy lifestyle? You do, but just know that willpower is not the same as belief. Willpower rates second behind beliefs, and if we change your beliefs, willpower flows easily and naturally!

Belief is a thousand times stronger than willpower because belief uses the unconscious mind to create behavior change with automation, while willpower uses the conscious mind to create behavior with force. And that's the goal of BLISS™, to change your beliefs about training and eating at the molecular level!

THE DOG WHISPERER

I love watching Caesar Milan from *The Dog Whisperer* whip frenzied, uncontrollable dogs into shape. Why? Because I learned one of the most valuable lessons from him – break the pattern, and start a new, fresh pattern with a change in energy.

That's what Caesar does when he works with a troubled dog – he breaks their current behavior pattern, quickly, before the dog can react, and puts a new one in its place. He breaks the 'Pavlov's dog' thing. The dog can no longer react to that which is no longer there. (Ever wonder why the dog sometimes looks confused or *de-fused* when he's around? Because they're on new territory, and the rules have changed.)

That's what I want for you, to put you on new turf, so to speak. This can be uncomfortable for awhile. After all, we've had these beliefs for many years. We can look at them on paper and see how they obviously have been limiting us. They've been like a suit of armor that we wear every day – protecting, yes, but heavy and constraining. And many times, there's no enemy left to protect us against! But we still think our beliefs continue to serve us on some level. They've kept us safe (if you don't try, you'll never have to fail), maintained the status quo (we don't risk changing our relationships) or kept us small (I don't want to be noticed). Whatever the reason, it's time to get brave and shed that suit of armor and feel light, confident and in control once again!

MY BELIEF MAP

I was brought up in a traditional family. In the '70s, girls were expected to do the cooking and cleaning, and to finish school and marry a nice guy. And while I did my best to fulfill these expectations and make my parents happy, I always felt that there must be more to life than that.

Then I found weight training and everything changed. I suddenly loved my new life and the freedom and creativity I had, and I even enjoyed throwing the female-gender-stereotypes right out the door. It was what I needed to let me live life on my terms.

I began to realize how much my beliefs had held me back, beliefs about what women were supposed to do and what was expected of them! But what I didn't realize was that these beliefs were hand-me-downs! There was no real basis for them in my life, yet they were *running my life*! They were subconscious and it was only when I paused to look long enough that I started to look at things differently.

UPDATING YOUR BELIEFS

We are always reviewing and changing our beliefs, and this is how it's supposed to be. How many of you believed in Santa Claus as a child? How many of you have a very different idea of romantic love or marriage now than you did when you were sixteen? How about parenting? Are your ideas about what it takes to be a good parent the same ideas you had when you began the process?

Case in point, our beliefs change as we continue to grow and gather new experiences. They change as we gather new information from books and the media. As things ring true for us we adopt or embrace new beliefs. We aren't consciously thinking about this fact, or calling it such, but it is what we all do.

The beauty of seeing that we are always changing beliefs, and acknowledging that we don't really do this consciously, is realizing that if we're doing it anyway then we can become *conscious belief changers*. We can consciously choose and embrace beliefs that support the feelings and behaviors we want to have and the life we want to make for ourselves.

Some people practice the power of positive thinking, repeating mantras hoping to have them sink into their unconscious and become habits. Others use the practice of logical thinking. Still others might try hypnosis, hoping to have someone else hypnotize them into believing that cigarettes really do taste like lima beans! I can think of better ways!

WHAT'S YOUR STORY?

For years, I've lectured to at-risk youth and I'm always learning something from these teens. Many of them come from tough backgrounds and are often struggling with addiction and issues of abuse and abandonment.

I recall one young lady in one of the classes who was rebellious from the get-go. Whenever I would talk about starting an exercise regime, she said she couldn't because of one thing or another. Clean eating was another issue, and she had a dozen reasons why she couldn't do it. She was the ultimate victim of her life, and nothing seemingly went her way, and she insisted that nothing was her fault (or her responsibility).

At one point I was getting annoyed with her constant roadblocks, but then I realized what was really happening and I settled into it: this poor young woman was just a victim of learned behavior. Somewhere along the way, she was taught that everything was outside of her control and that there was no use trying anything, because she was not in control of her own life. She had given up her power (I'm guessing from a very early age) and started making excuses for why she couldn't do anything because it was everyone else's fault, not hers.

She had created a story in her head, and it was a learned behavior that was likely passed down from her parents or caregivers. She was the victim here and she wasn't going to budge from that belief. (Victims have it easy because by blaming something or someone else for their lack of success, they don't have to take responsibility.)

Like this young woman, we all create our own reality by the stories in our heads, those hamster-like stories we replay over and over again... they're *not reality*, they're our *stories*. But like this young woman, many of us can't see the forest for the trees. But that's where you have to really be honest with yourself if you want to truly change and live the life you deserve!

As mentioned earlier, my husband and I were struggling with issues in our relationship, and it's no wonder. I unconsciously rehearsed in my head all the ways he upset me. Let's see... he was harsh / critical / overbearing / silent.... Or how about this... he never listened to me / wanted to talk / appreciated all I did.... Sound familiar?

It wasn't until I learned to *change my inner story* that our relationship truly transformed. Instead of looking at the negative traits, I reminded myself how kind / funny / handsome / supportive he was. Pretty soon, everything started to shift. And I realized I hadn't married the wrong person at all. In fact, he was (and still is) the man of my dreams, the one I envisioned years ago. I just needed to shift my story and focus on all the great stuff we had. Pretty soon, all that moved to the forefront and we lived from that place – fresh, exciting, empowering again!

You can do the same with training and healthy eating. But you must dig down, and take responsibility for *everything* you do. You must be willing to own it all. And remember this is *your* journey, *your* work, no one else's. This is YOU changing YOU because you care about you! And when you start to shift and change, an amazing thing starts to happen: others will start shifting as well. That's because change in one always creates change in another, because that invisible web of energy connects everything and everyone together, kind of like ripples in the ocean.

We need to really look deeply (and with courage), into two distinct areas: exercise and eating!

IT'S YOUR TURN –
CHANGING YOUR LIMITING BELIEFS

When I take on a new client, I always ask what their goals are. Usually it's the same thing: to lose weight and to look and feel better. While I write down what they're saying, more importantly, I'm making mental notes about how they're sitting and other subtle body clues, because I've learned that a person's story is written in their bodies.

So ask yourself this question – *what do you really feel about exercise and clean eating?* If you're like some of us, you just can't wait to get to the gym. You jump out of bed and into your training clothes, grab your water bottle and you're off! Sadly, this isn't the case with everyone. A lot of people would rather hit the snooze button than go exercise. The thought of training just looks like another to-do item in their already busy day. Is this true, or is this what they have come to believe is true?

Have you ever said any of the following things to yourself?

"I hate to exercise."

"I've tried to lose weight before and it's never worked."

"It's going to hurt."

"I don't want to feel in denial of food all the time, it's too painful."

"I don't have the time."

"I don't have the genetics."

"I don't have the money."

"She's lucky, she can do it because she has more … (support / money / time)."

These are all stories that you tell yourself, and you need to ask yourself why. Is it because you fear success, or you don't want to challenge family members? Is it a way to lay blame and to not take responsibility?

Can you turn it around? What if you got excited by the process? What if you saw exercise as *empowering*? What if you knew you would live a pain-free life because of your efforts?

CREATING A NEW BELIEF MAP

So how can we dismember our old beliefs and update our Belief Map? Here are a few tried and true tools I've used with my clients (and myself) for years.

- CHANGE YOUR STORY, CHANGE YOUR LIFE: We already touched on this but it bears repeating – *You must change your story about who you are.* If you say, "It'll never happen, I can't do it, I'm no good, I don't like to exercise, I'm not going to stick with it," then guess what – you're right!

    The Universe hears your inner whispers and doesn't differentiate between a good thought or a bad one – it delivers regardless. I'm living proof of this, and so are you.

- CHANGE YOUR LANGUAGE: Instead of saying, "I hate to sweat / hurt / train...", try looking at it from another angle. Try saying, "I love feeling tight and toned after my session, and I love watching my body transform day after day." Get inspired!

- MAKE A DECISION: When it comes to creating a successful fitness or health program, it must be *your decision.* If you're there because your doctor told you to be there, or your husband or children urged you to go, you're not likely to stick with it. That's because, in essence, you've given your power away to others. It has to be *your* decision.

- WALK AS IF....: Whether it's to lose 20 pounds or tighten your abs, you must envision what you're going to look like. This stokes the training fires like nothing else and helps bring it closer to you. *Walk as if* and *feel* like you already have it, and the Universe will serve it up to you (with some elbow grease from you!). This works in all areas of life – finances, love relationships, career… everything.

- FIND YOUR INNER GRRRR! A young client of mine who was a competitive rock climber explained where she got her inner motivation to train. She loved to train, and she couldn't wait to get into the gym. She called that burning feeling in her solar plexus her inner grrrr.

  Do you feel that inner grrrr in your body? For me, when I'm excited about a new possibility, I always feel expansive and fluttery in my solar plexus. So before you embark on my BLISS™ Program, check in with your body – do you feel expansive and excited or do you feel tight and constricted? This is your body's inner wisdom, its emotional guidance system at work, and you need to listen to it. If you feel like you're expanding, great! Then you're on the right track. If, however, you feel like you're contracting, then you need to look at your inner beliefs and re-create ones that are uplifting.

- READ OTHER PEOPLE'S STORIES. Perhaps my story is one that inspires you. Or perhaps you have a favourite fitness personality you've come to respect. Whoever it is, find something or someone that inspires you! Read fitness magazines and the success stories, programs and menu plans within them. I always have a copy of *Oxygen, Women's Health* or *Fitness Rx* on my nightstand or some health-related book that I can thumb through to keep me motivated and inspired. I've been doing this for 30 years and it keeps my fires stoked!

- CUT OUT THE NAY SAYERS. Unfortunately, there are people who will try to derail your intentions (friends and family, listen up!). As you get better / happier / stronger, others may feel anxious about your new-found health regime. Know that it's their issue, not yours. Don't make yourself small for anyone. It serves no one – not them, and certainly not you.

• GET MOMENTUM. Nike had it right with their now-famous tag line, *just do it*. You're not going to create the life of your dreams by sitting on your tush. Start moving and things will naturally get drawn to you. Opportunities will arise. You'll meet someone who can help you on your path, or you'll read something that will inspire you or answer that burning question you've had all these years. Momentum creates opportunity in action.

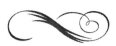

FIVE

Food and YOU!

A big part of the success of my BLISS™ Training Method is its approach to eating, both in the physical aspect (calories, portions, etc.), and the emotional aspect. So take a moment and consider how you eat. Do you eat poorly when you are stressed or get too little sleep, or when you're perhaps having too much fun? Do you eat differently when you travel? On weekends? When you're alone? Do you lack planning in your meals?

You need to understand that *what goes on between your ears is what's opening the lever to your jaw.* So if we can understand why we do things, we have the foundation for making lasting change. Let's take a closer look.

THE FIVE EATING STYLES –WHICH ARE YOU?

Research has found that there are 5 eating styles that derail our best attempts at eating well. Do you recognize yourself in any of these descriptors? Research also shows that if you can see it, you can change it. So let's see which one(s) of these you associate with.

- THE PROCRASTINATOR: You want to make changes but you continue to come up with excuses. You want to wait until that long weekend is over, or until your job settles in, or until life slows down. But life never slows down. Many of us are waiting for that magical push to get us started, but it rarely comes. This sets you up for failure.

  So set yourself up for success by taking small steps. Print your grocery list at the beginning of the week and put a copy of it on your fridge. Stock healthy snacks at home or at work. Keep a water bottle with you at all times. Small shifts create small successes that can make you feel more and more competent, and will not overwhelm you and cause you to derail your efforts. A Procrastinator needs only to take the first step. So make it small, and make it stick. Your mantra is to *get started and keep going.*

- THE EMOTIONAL EATER: Is food your comfort when you're stressed, guilty, angry or lonely? Or is food the enemy, something to be controlled or restricted in times of stress? Do you binge, feel guilty, restrict, feel worse, binge and repeat? Every day bring stresses, and to continually use food as a coping mechanism, you're in for a lifetime of anxiety, guilt, low self-esteem and poor health.

  It's necessary to know your triggers, then you have to find other ways to deal with these emotions: journal, talk out loud, cry, go for a run. Face it head on, name it, say it out loud and you've shifted the pattern. And choose another behavior: if you're lonely, and you want to grab some food, instead call a friend, or write a list of what you're grateful about. Change the behavior, change the pattern, change your life. Look at food as fuel, health-building, a chance to positively change the structure of your cells. Use it in a new way, to see it in a new light. Your mantra is to *call it what it is, OUT LOUD. (I'm lonely, angry, sad....)*

- THE REACTIVE EATER: Lack of structure is the villain here, due to lack of awareness of the amount of food consumed over the day. The reactive eater eats in the car, grabs calories from vending machines or is so busy, she forgets to eat. This leads to missed meals, and grabbing whatever is available when hunger eventually consumes you.

  First, don't eat while doing other things. This will make you focus in and be aware of what you're eating. *Second,* plan your meals. A proactive eater is more likely to make healthy choices, less likely to skip meals and will be able to listen to the subtle clues of hunger and react better at the time. Your mantra is to *plan your meals for the day, and eat without doing something else at the time.*

- THE PORTION DISTORTIONIST: This eater doesn't understand how much food her body actually needs. She oscillates between overeating (whether it's healthy food or not), and restricting to maintain a certain weight. Often we're taught to clean our plates, or you just got accustomed to eating larger portions. Remember, a protein portion is the size of your palm,

Another group of hard-working women who transformed themselves over a 3-month period. Shapely, toned and sexy! Whenever we get together, I always bring dessert! Usually chocolate cake (my favourite!)

a grain portion is half a cup (measure it out, it's quite small!), and a serving of fruits or veggies is the size of a tennis ball. That's it. That's one meal.

Did you know today's generation doesn't even know what an 8-ounce drink really is? A serving of cheese is the size of a pair of dice. Once you figure out the real size of something, you'll likely find that you're eating 2 to 3 times the servings you need. Throw out the dinner plate and use a salad or side plate as your visual guide. Now you're back to where we were 20 years ago. Your mantra: *I only need a side-plate sized meal to satisfy all my caloric needs.*

- THE EVENING EATER: For these eaters, they consume most of their calories from dinner on through to night time. Remember,

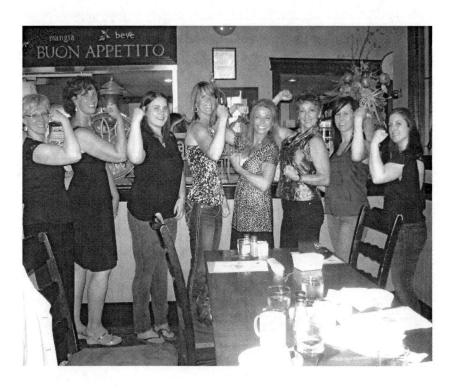

it's not just how many calories but when you consume them as well. Calories consumed earlier in the day, when our metabolism is naturally higher, can be burned off easier. As the sun sets, so too does our metabolism, and it just can't burn off the food as efficiently. Hence 100 calories late at night acts like 200 calories!

Planning is key to success for the evening eater. Start the day with breakfast, write out your meals to ensure you've eaten at least 3 before dinner, then one more at dinner and you're set. That's it. Your Mantra: *I'm eating a good breakfast, and I've planned for a snack and for a lunch meal.*

You can't change something if you don't recognize it. So take a good look at your eating style. Once you identify your type, you're on your way to winning the battle of harmful eating for good!

HOW TO TELL THE DIFFERENCE BETWEEN PHYSICAL AND EMOTIONAL HUNGER

The BLISS™ Training Method teaches us that there are some very distinct differences between physical and emotional hunger, and we need to differentiate between them for lasting success.

- Physical hunger builds up gradually, starting with a tiny grumble in the stomach, growing to full-blown hunger pangs. Emotional hunger develops suddenly.
- With physical hunger, you can wait if you have to. Emotional hunger seems to demand immediate satisfaction.

- Physical hunger usually appears about three hours after the last meal or snack. Emotional hunger can happen anytime.
- Physical hunger is a general desire for food. Emotional hunger is a desire for specific food.
- After eating for physical hunger, the hunger goes away. After emotional hunger, it persists.
- After eating for physical hunger, you feel satisfied. After eating for emotional reasons, you feel guilty.

HOW TO SHIFT FROM EMOTIONAL EATING TO REAL EATING

While most people think there is an emotional link to eating, few of us channel back to our childhood to find it. Rather, we cite reasons like, "It just tastes good," or "I've always eaten that way." Let's shift from being unconscious to being conscious.

STEP 1:
BECOME AWARE OF YOUR EATING BEHAVIORS

While you may like ice cream because it tastes good, digging deeper uncovers more… For one of my clients it reminded her of being at the summer house when she was a little girl. For guys, drinking beer might bring them back to those rugby days when all the guys hung out after the game and enjoyed the post-game party, even long after their playing days have ended.

First, let's try something called eating exclusively. That means when you eat, you do nothing but eat. Studies show that TV time correlates highly with weight gain and obesity, likely because you are unaware of how much you're eating, and you tie munching in front of the TV with reward and relaxation.

Second, you have to eat slowly. There are several reasons for this:

- When you eat fast, your tummy can't signal your brain fast enough to notify when it's full, so you keep eating even when you've had enough.

- Also, when we choose foods that are easy to chew and have a low energy density (man-made foods, breads, pasta), you plow through them quickly and effortlessly, again, leading to over-eating. Plus, their caloric-dense nature ensures more calories per bite.

So chew high density foods that fill you up and force you to eat slowly. For example, a cup of broccoli requires more chewing and more digesting time, and is a high density food given its fiber nature, and is sure to fill you up more than a cup of ice cream.

Third, keep a *food journal*. Onerous? Sometimes. Necessary? YES, if only for a while (2 to 3 months minimum). It should include not just your food, but also records your thoughts and emotions. A journal is a real wake-up call and allows you to see the emotional triggers and links that have run your life for years.

STEP 2:
WATCH OUT FOR YOUR EMOTIONAL TRIGGERS

Emotional eating doesn't just happen by chance, there's always a trigger. So do some detective work. What pushes your emotional eating buttons? As you move through the list, know that triggers generally fall into one of four categories: feelings, places, people or events.

Stress	Overwork	Buffets
Loneliness	Overwhelm	Restaurants
Boredom	Fatigue / exhaustion	Food in the kitchen
Anger	Financial challenges	Smell of food
Frustration	Relationship challenges	Sight of food
Sadness	Parties	Time of day
Feeling ignored	Holidays	Time of month
Feeling unloved	Weather	Television

STEP 3:
STOP NEGATIVE PATTERNS WHEN THEY HAPPEN

When you become aware of an urge to eat inappropriately, it's an important moment of decision. Awareness gives you the chance to have a conversation with yourself in those critical moments before you act. Remind yourself, "I could always eat this later, but for now, let me think about what eating this might do to me."

The important thing is to stop, pause, and think before you eat. That gives you time to ask yourself some important questions:

- Am I thinking about eating because I'm physically hungry or for another reason?
- If it's not for physical hunger, then why am I thinking about eating this?

- What will be the long-term consequences if I eat this?
- What will be my rewards for saying no to this?
- Is eating this going to move me closer to or further away from my goals?
- Is eating this worth it?

Personally, I always look at the after-effects: Do I want to eat this processed, unnatural food if it's going to become every part of every cell in my body – my muscles, brain, lungs and skin? Then I ask myself, How will I look and feel after I've eaten this? How will my tummy look in that tight dress of mine? Better still, will doing this make me feel proud or will I have let myself down? It's worth questioning.

STEP 4:
REPLACE OLD EMOTIONAL EATING BEHAVIORS
WITH MORE CONSTRUCTIVE ALTERNATIVES

There are always constructive ways to satisfy any feeling. It's not about the food, it's about the feeling you thought you'd get from eating. So what are you really hungry for? Companionship? Love? Happiness?

The key is learning that you can't recapture that feeling from food, in fact, you usually feel worse (guilt / shame / defeat) after eating. So the trick is to 'put a chink in the chain' and break the pattern.

- Brush your teeth
- Do 10 pushups
- Turn off the TV
- Journal
- Mediate

- Go for a 30-minute walk
- Read
- Call a friend.

Whatever you do, remember, *if you keep doing what you're doing, you'll keep getting what you got.* So you must change your behavior by replacing it with something else to break those neurological pathways that are laid down and have been reinforced for years! Just trying to take away the offending behavior is usually not successful (nature abhors a vacuum!). So try a new tactic, make a new behavior and you're on the right path!

STEP 5:
CREATE NEW BELIEFS ABOUT FOOD
AND THEN PRACTICE, PRACTICE, PRACTICE!

We often think that people who can stick to their clean eating without swaying have superhuman strength and motivation. While it's true that this is part of it, really, it's about having established and implemented over and over again a new way of eating, and a new way of thinking about food. With time, you too will eventually shift your thinking about food and help set your new behaviors in stone.

When I was competing, I had to drastically change how I ate. It was a tough go at first, but eventually I learned this new style of eating. Now I think it's odd to eat large dinners, and to eat bread and butter. My largest meal now is always a late lunch, with dinner being a small portion or a collection of healthy snacks.

If you believe that hunger pangs are negative, or painful, then you'll never lose weight and keep it off. If you believe exercise is something you *have to do* rather than something you *get to do*, you won't stick with it. If you believe healthy eating is about denial and not having fun, then you'll never stay lean. Change your perspective around food. Create a new language, and thus a new understanding, around food.

- Food is fuel
- Food is my best medicine
- Food stokes the fire of metabolism
- Lean protein will create tight, shapely muscle and strong bones
- When I eat clean, I feel light, tight and in control
- When I feel hungry, I know I'm burning fat
- When I eat fibrous veggies, I'm cleaning out my body and releasing nasty chemicals
- When I eat organic, I'm keeping my body clean and toxin-free
- It's possible to eat well when I'm travelling.

UPDATE YOUR BELIEF MAP

Remember, it's hard to just say no to an old belief or habit, you need to replace old, negative thoughts with something powerful, uplifting and different! Choose perhaps just two or three to focus on and build from there.

This is also a powerful exercise to do in all aspects of your life – love, finances, career and family. Please remember that this is your life in the making. You are not here by default, and you are not supposed to live your life by default. You are free to choose and live as you please. You are a co-creator of your world.

CREATING YOUR NEW BELIEF MAP

Write down your *current* *beliefs* about exercise & eating.	Now *re-write* them! Go for it!
Here's an example:	
When I feel hunger pangs, it's uncomfortable, unnatural.	*When I feel hungry, my body is burning fat, and I'm getting leaner every day!*
I don't want to train because I hate feeling sore all the time.	*When I feel sore, it means I'm shaping and toning my muscles, and I'm revving up my metabolism by adding shapely muscle!*

YOUR TURN...

1. _____   _____

   _____   _____

2. _____   _____

   _____   _____

3. _____

4. _____

5. _____

6. _____

7. _____

8. _____

Every woman has a story, and every woman is a success story in herself. I always say that training and clean eating is the greatest act of self-love you can practice. We owe it to ourselves!

9. _____

_____

10. _____

_____

Okay. Now that we've cleared away the cobwebs, and put some fresh goals and beliefs in place, let's move on. **NOTE:** Remember to write your GOALS and BELIEFS onto your **BLISS™ FOCUS CARDS** and carry them with you! You'll find your downloadable **FOCUS CARDS** on your on-line **WORKOUT PAGE.**

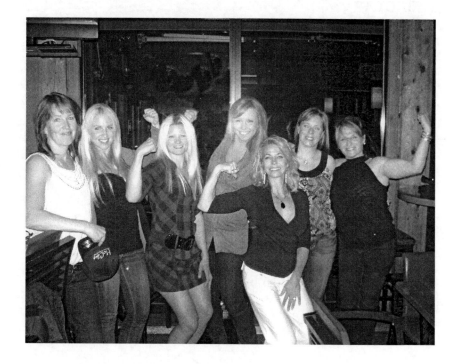

SIX

Gathering Your Tools

OK. Before we get started, let's take stock of what we'll need before
we begin our training.

GYM GEAR

- WATER BOTTLE: be prepared to fill it at least 2 times! And
  make sure it's 750 ml or 1 litre
- FULL LENGTH PANTS: shorts can be uncomfortable, especially when laying on some of the benches
- GOOD SHOES: solid running shoes with support
- PERIPHERALS: workout gloves (personal choice), lifting belt
  and/or wraps (personal choice), towel, hair band (yep, tie it
  back)
- IPOD: If you must, use it for your cardio for now. Remember
  your lifting will now take on a meditative quality from here on
  in. Being present is so important in the art of body (and life)
  transformation.

USE A FOOD DIARY

Yep, you're going to count calories and you're going to write them down. I can hear the protests, but believe me when I say this is an extremely important part of BLISS™, and one I won't waver on. It's not forever, but it is for the next few weeks. Studies show that with journaling, there is an 80% greater success rate in people who write down what they eat than in those who do not.

NOTE: You'll find blank food journals on the program's web page, but you're free to use your own.

If you're the kind of person that is mystified by the lack of weight loss, truly mystified, then calorie counting is a good idea. Because in my experience, most people underestimate how much they eat, and only when they start measuring their portions and counting up calories can they truly see that they are over-consuming or using too-large portions. However, if you're truly honest with yourself and you know where you're slipping up with your eating, then no need for counting calories. Just stop the offending behaviour.

I always like to see people return to calorie counting, even if they've done it a lot in the past, because getting re-acquainted with calories can be important. And some foods (and packaging) have changed over the years, so we need to get re-acquainted with it all.

Counting calories doesn't have to be tedious, but it does require diligence, at least for a little while, anyway. Once you get the hang of it, you'll be able to eyeball something and know within seconds how many calories are in that meal and you won't need your reference book anymore.

For successfully counting calories, you'll need a few tools:
- MEASURING UTENSILS – measuring spoons, measuring cup

and a scale. Sound onerous? It can be, but truly, some people don't know how much 4 ounces is, or how little 1/2 cup truly is.

- CALORIE COUNTER BOOK – found in most book stores. My favourite is *The Biggest Loser – Complete Calorie Counter*. It's fast and easy to use. Or you can use any good counter found on the Internet. I like www.fitday.com

- FOOD JOURNAL – Studies show that diets are 80% more successful with people who write things down. It makes you accountable, you see the holes in your eating, and you think twice about cheating. Either use a paper journal, or try an on-line calorie counter program – check out *sparkpeople.com*, *thecaloriecounter.com*, or *fitday.com* (my personal favourite).

- BODY MEASUREMENTS – *weight, body fat* and *tape measure*. How can you know how far you've come unless you know where you came from? And nothing creates a positive environment like seeing your success on paper. (Your Body Measurement Sheet is included in the program.)

You'll want to do your body fat too (as well as your weight) but not everyone has their own body fat tool at home. If not, your local gym likely has one. I use the **Omron HBF-306 Body Fat Analyzer** which retails for about $40 and is very simple to use. You can buy them online. Whichever one you use, always use that same one or results will vary. You want to aim for 20 to 25% body fat. If you're above 30%, we'll focus on getting it lower.

TAKE PHOTOS

For photos, take a picture of yourself in your bathing suit from three angles – front, side and back (it's all explained in your **Body Measurements and Photo Sheet** found on your **Workout Page**). Save these to your binder. Trust me, this step is very important. It's uncomfortable, but when you start seeing results, you'll truly appreciate having done so.

TRACKING YOUR PROGRESS

You'll be writing down what you do every day including sets, reps, weights, cardio and stretching on your **Tracking Sheet** which you'll find in each Training Package. Don't forget this step! It's an important part of the process, and not only solidifies your commitment, it also ensures progressive, continual success, as you'll be needing to change exercises, weights, reps, sets on an on-going basis. This is *progressive* weight training.

SEVEN

Stepping Inside a Gym

For the first few weeks of the program, you can train at home if you wish, with minimal equipment. But eventually, you'll need to progress to a gym.

Stepping inside a gym is a different experience for many women. If you're like me, you love this part of the program. But for many women, it's alienating and intimidating. Not to worry. Everyone has their own comfort level, but just remember this: no one's really watching you. They're too busy doing their work (hopefully!).

TRAINING AT HOME – BEWARE THE PITFALLS

Many women have no option but to train at home, given family responsibilities, distance or finances. But in my experience, you have to be really diligent to get a good workout at home. I always say the drop-out rate for training at home is high because there are all sorts of distractions. As well, you may be doing the exercises wrong and no one can correct you (so please watch the videos closely to ensure you're using the proper form).

CHOOSING A GYM

Years ago, gyms really varied in what they offered in the way of equipment, fees and trainers. But these days, almost every gym is equal in that respect, with a few variances. It's a competitive business, so they're forced to stay on top of things. Whatever your choice, don't be dazzled with a lot of equipment. When it gets right down to it, you can get an extremely effective workout with 3 sets of dumbbells, some barbells, a few solid benches and a few choice machines. I've trained in gyms the size of your average living room when nothing else was available, and I did just fine.

CHOOSING A TRAINER

The 8-Week BLISS™ Body Makeover Program will be all the trainer you need, but sometimes it's wise to check in with a trainer if you're unsure, or if you want to make sure you're doing the exercises right. All I can say is that while you hope all trainers are equal, they are not. Check for length of experience (these days, you can get a trainer certificate in 3 easy weekends). Better yet, check them out – do they walk the walk? Do they look like they train? Do they have the physique you emulate? Nothing ticks me off more than someone not leading by example. If they teach it, they should live it, so check them out!

Do They Walk the Walk? Remember, there's no substitute for experience. I always say **the proof is in the pudding**. Whatever we do in life, whatever our vocation, in order for others to believe in us, we must lead by example. *We gotta walk the walk!* I'm always amazed when I see trainers spout off about the benefits of eating clean, only to see them scarfing down some fast-food travesty behind the counter!

Please! If you see that, run! Do NOT give that person your money or your time!

If I were overweight and ate McDonald's all day, would you still be buying this book? I don't think so. I try to live the life every day, as best I can. Sure, we all fall off the healthy bandwagon once in a while, but the point is, we get back up! And I've fallen a thousand times, and gotten back up. It's called life. It's not about perfection, it's about *being real*. So be careful who you follow and listen to. Getting in awesome shape requires diligence and focus. It MUST be a lifestyle, and in fitness, you can clearly see with your eyes if that person walks the walk!

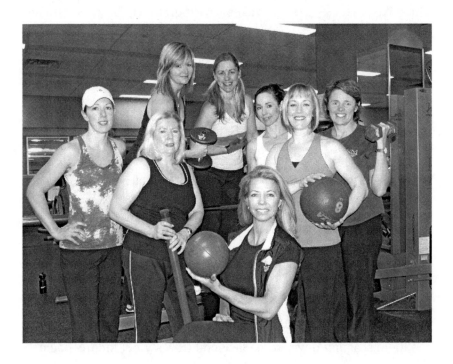

EIGHT

BLISS™ Training Tips

Real weight training is both a physical and a spiritual practice, but most people don't really understand this aspect at the start. But with practice and focus, you'll learn to lift the BLISS™ way, with intention and clarity. At this point, I want you to put away your IPod and focus in silence. Most people zone out with an iPod. I want you to learn to zone in.

- WARRIOR STANCE: When you lift, take the warrior stance – head and shoulders up and back, knees slightly bent and shoulder-width apart, core area tight and back straight. Imagine the power of the Earth coming up through your feet and into your body. Stay connected.
- ZONE IN: Get into your Zen – close your eyes, breathe deeply, and go into your quiet zone. Envision what you want your body to look and feel like. Which muscles are you working?
- LIFT: Envision being inside your muscles. See the sinewy

Me and my group of hard-working gals at the gym pause for a photo!

fibers laying row upon row. See the strength and vitality there. Get into the muscle. Now lift and envision your muscle expanding and contracting, drawing in the life force all around you. Enjoy the feeling of power coursing through your body. Be grateful for the ability to train.

- SPEED: When lifting, move at an average pace (even this can change according to your goals, but for now, let's keep it simple). Try for a two-second count up and down.

- BREATHING: Exhale on exertion, so when you come to the hardest part of the lift (i.e., curling that dumbbell up to your chest), breathe out, and breathe in upon return. Think like a Jedi Master – they yell (expel air) when they are breaking a board or performing a huge lift.

- MAKE EVERY SET A WORK OF ART: You need to focus in, *see* your muscles working, envision them changing, and focus on the work at hand. You are carving and creating your body and your world. Enjoy it!

- REST INTERVALS: Don't get too caught up in counting the minutes here, but aim to take a break between sets for around 30 seconds to a full 90 seconds or more. It all depends on how hard you work. If you lift heavy, you need more time. If you want to do a circuit style, you naturally want to keep the rest to a minimum. I aim for about 45 to 60 seconds break between lifts.

- FINDING YOUR WORKING WEIGHT: Remember, you've got to lift large to get small and tight. But for the first few weeks, we're going to have you lift moderate weights, in order to build up your strength and tolerance for exercise. You'll find all this information in your *Training Packages.*

- APPLYING THE PROGRESSIVE OVERLOAD PRINCIPAL: As you work through the program, you'll be steadily increasing your weights to support the progressive overload theory, which ensures continual improvement in shape, strength and tone, and with few plateaus. This theory also applies to your cardio workout so be sure to gradually increase the difficulty of your cardio.

NINE

How to Stay Motivated!

Ask any successful athlete or anyone that's made huge shifts in their health and they'll all say the same thing: getting there is one job, but staying there is a whole other job. This can truly be the toughest part of it all, but I promise you that, if you feel *truly motivated*, your new lifestyle will become a sheer pleasure. It won't feel like work at all!

So how can you stay motivated day after day? Here are a few tools that I've used for years.

- PUT UP PICTURES: When I first started training, I stuck up pictures of my favourite male and female competitors all over the walls. I would look at their pictures while training because they inspired me to keep going! Go through fitness magazines and cut out pictures of women you admire. Put them on your fridge, in your car, at work or wherever you can see them often.

At my Advanced Workshop for Competitors (left to right) Leanne La Prairie, me, Deanna Pfeifer, Lesley Arnold and Teresa Touhy.

There's peace in knowing other women have gone before you, and if they can do it, so can you!

- MEDITATE / VISUALIZE: One extremely important aspect of success is the ability to envision your course and stay on track. This is where meditation comes into play big time! Don't worry about the how-to of meditation, it needn't be complicated. I practice it every day, first a.m. and at night before I go to bed. We'll look at this in more depth later, but just know that meditation is one of the quickest and surest ways of reaching deep into the subconscious where all change originates. Remember, meditation is not only done sitting on the floor with eyes closed... I do it all the time while shopping, driving and training! It's all in your Training Packages!

- LEAF THROUGH THE MAGAZINES: I always have a pile of fitness magazines by my bedside table that I leaf through every

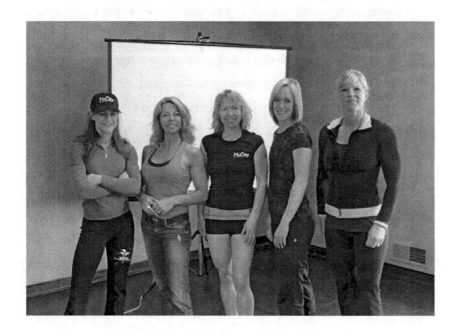

night: *Oxygen, Women's Health, Men's Health* and *Inside Fitness.* It's like filling up the tank (my mind) before going to bed each night. It keeps me inspired!

- GO TO SHOWS: Every year, we attend fitness and body building shows. I always walk away highly charged and ready to hit the training hard the next day! It's a great source of motivation for me.

- BOOKS: I have a host of exercise and clean eating books in my home office. I will often look through them when I'm taking a break, or when I feel I need some words of wisdom. They remind me of all the great mentors and teachers who have gone before me. I always get inspired by my favourite health authors: Sam Graci, Crystal Andrus, Cory Holly, Michael Colgan and Tom Venuto.

- CHANGE YOUR THINKING, CHANGE YOUR LIFE! If a new client starts with, "I hate to exercise," I tell them to go home. I'm not trying to be mean, but how can I help them with anything if they've shut the gates in their own mind? However, if they're willing to try to open up to the possibilities and to challenge their thinking, then I will certainly do all I can to support their new lifestyle.

I'm going to repeat my mantra again: *health and wellness is an inside job.* If you wish to achieve anything – health, career, love, wealth – you need to change how you think before you step into the gym in order to have true success. Because how you truly feel about training and eating creates the undercurrent that will either enhance or sabotage your efforts. Change your thinking, change your life!

DEBUNKING THE MYTHS (AGAIN!)

It surprises me that the old myths still abound. By now, you know after reading my book that there are no myths when it comes to training and eating for women, only hype and misinformation. But let's go through them again, in case you missed some of them.

Q: If I eat too much protein, will I put on too much muscle?

A: Competitors and athletes wish it could be that simple! You need to lift heavy and with consistency to build muscle, and even then, it's a slow build, with most women seeing maybe 3 to 5 pounds of new muscle in a year (if they're lucky!). We'll touch on what kinds of protein and in what amounts you need to eat in the program.

Q: Can I spot reduce?

A: This is the most often heard question out there. In fact, even those of us that know better still fall prey to it: "I over-indulged last night, I better go work my abs." We know better, right? The muscle does not own the fat around it, so to get fat off your thighs / abs / butt, you must tend to your nutrition. Period. Weight training will create the shapely muscle underneath, but it won't burn the fat off that specific area.

Q: But if I train with weights, won't I get too bulky? I gain muscle easily.

A: No, and no. You won't get too bulky and you don't really gain muscle fast. It's physically impossible for women to do so. We just don't have the amount of muscle-building hormones that men have. When the scale goes up, and your clothes feel tighter, it's due to over-hydration – you've torn your muscles and your body draws in more water and nutrients to heal (this can last for weeks). If in doubt, use a body fat device and you'll find that while your weight may go up, it's not body fat: it's due to minimal muscle growth and lots of excess water.

Q: Can I speed up my metabolism?

A: Yes and no. Genetics certainly play a part here, but we can speed up the metabolism by eating whole, unprocessed foods, increasing our protein intake and drinking more water. And of course, we need to add in weight training (muscle burns fat, so the more muscle, the more fat-burning ability) and some cardio. We go over this in your BLISS™ Program.

Q: Isn't it best to use high reps and lower weights?

A: Boy, let's turn this one around right away! The whole basis of the BLISS™ Program is to lift heavy and lift often. But many women are scared of this. Don't be! You'll soon learn that the more you lift and the less reps you do, the faster the results – faster shaping and toning, a faster metabolism and you'll get smaller and tighter. You gotta lift BIG to get small! You'll see!

Q: Is it true that the more cardio I do, the more weight I'll lose? And long and slow is best?

A: With the BLISS™ training method, we'll actually do less cardio and lose more fat weight! That's where high intensity interval training (HIIT) comes in over long slow distance (LSD). I'll show you how it's done!

Q: Don't women have to train differently than men?

A: Nope. Intensity is intensity. And your framework will lay down muscle according to your female make-up and build – your ligament insertions, bone structure, and joint capsules all dictate how you look. If you don't look like a man now, how are you going to look like a man when you add on shapely, sexy muscle?

Q: But if I squat, won't I get a big butt?

A: No. In fact, you'll get a big butt if you don't squat! The glutes are a muscle too and they definitely need exercise. Our ever-expanding butts are due to fat (and inactivity). Squatting will make it tight and firm!

Q: If I can't work out often and hard enough, should I even bother?

A: Yes! The general rule for weight loss is to do cardio 4 to 5 times a week for a minimum of 20 minutes, and weight training 3 or more times a week. Some people simply don't have the time to work out much and think that if they can't do all of that, why do ANY of it? Remember, any exercise is better than no exercise, even if it's only a 15-minute walk. Besides, being physically active is proven to reduce stress and make you healthier.

Q: If I'm not sore the next day, does it mean I didn't work out hard enough?

A: Muscle soreness is caused by tiny tears in the muscle fibers (NOT lactic acid). While some soreness is expected, being sore for days after your workout most likely means you overdid it, but yes, you do need to feel some soreness! That means you've challenged your muscles. Sorry, but the *no pain, no gain* motto does apply. In time, you'll feel tight rather than sore, and when you do, you'll love the feeling! But if you up the ante, you will feel more sore for a while, that's called the progressive overload principle at work.

Q: But I'm too old for it to make a real difference, don't you think?
A: Oh boy, I can see we've got a lot of work to do. Let's park that myth at the door right now! Perhaps you're using it as an excuse for a lifetime of non-activity. Nothing can be further from the truth. Trust me! I've said it before and I'll say it again: In my experience, *weight training is the only sport where you get better with age*! The ability to create a shapely, sexy physique gets easier with every lift. With continual lifting, your muscles age better, and their shape and tone get sharper and more refined. It's also easier to keep the weight off. Of course, if you stop, the benefits start reversing, as in all sports. But you're not going to stop, right?

FREQUENTLY ASKED QUESTIONS

Please feel welcome to ask me questions, and to ask any other trainer. We are here to help! Each of us had to learn from someone, and you can't progress if you are stuck with an un-answered question. Here are some typical questions I receive from new participants in my courses.

Q: When will the soreness go away?
A: I'll let you in on a little secret – the soreness never really goes

away, even for elite athletes, but it changes from all-out sore to the touch type of soreness to a nice feeling of tightness. Of course, if you take lots of time off, you have to get sore all over again (incentive to staying consistent!), but it's normal in the first few weeks to be really sore. If you're really sore, do the movements but at a lesser weight, and drink your water. It'll flush out the lactic acid and accumulating toxins.

Q: How do I know I'm training hard enough?

A: If you're sore or feeling tight, you're training hard enough. It's all a matter of degrees. If the next day you really don't feel anything, then you have to up the intensity.

Q: I'm a little pressed for time. Can I fit it all in 1 hour?

A: The first few weeks of the program are the longest, not because the workouts are long, but because you're just getting used to reading the workouts, getting a feel for the moves, and moving through things a bit slower. With time, things will speed up. Give yourself a chance to learn these new tools of yours.

Q: My weight isn't going down... what's wrong?

A: Patience! We all want so much to see that scale move down, but your body is trying to learn to do a whole bunch of new stuff all at once. And remember, your body may momentarily be overhydrating to help heal your newly trained muscles, so the scale isn't always a good representation of true fat loss, especially in the first few weeks.

Q: I want to get the fat off my abs. Will more ab work do the trick?

A: Remember what we said? There's no such thing as spot reducing. You'll see them pop out when you remove the layers of fat on top.

Q: If I miss some or all of a workout in one day, should I make up for it the next day?

A: Nope. Don't stack them up. Just move forward and continue to train that workout for that day only. Tomorrow's a new day.

Q: My strength really increased, but now after a few weeks I feel weaker. Why?

A: At first, your strength can increase quite dramatically, but after about 2 weeks, your body puts the brakes on as it tries to play catch up with its recuperative abilities. Pretty soon it'll all catch up to each other. Then your strength gains will be less dramatic but consistent with every workout.

Okay. I think I've said enough… are you ready to get started? Then let's head over to the **BLISS™ Workout Page** and start your **8-Week BLISS™ Body Makeover Program**. Go to www.mccoyfitness.ca and click on the **Karen's Book** icon. Put in the program password – *blissbody.*

Enjoy! And email me with any questions, ok? I'm here to help and support you in your journey. Send to karen@mccoyfitness.ca

The Party's Over – Now What?

It's been eight great weeks, and I know if you've followed the BLISS™ program, you've experienced success in many ways and on many levels. At this point, I'd love to hear from you. Please email me at karen@mccoyfitness.ca. And remember, every month I choose one lucky woman to profile for my **Best BLISS™ Body Contest**. More information is found on the program web site! Loads of prizes and more!

Let's take a look at your accomplishments.
- Did you make the necessary nutrition and lifestyle changes you learned in the BLISS™ program?
- How do your measurements stack up? Did they shift?
- How do you look? Are your clothes fitting better?
- How do you feel? Are you feeling more confident and powerful?
- What other changes have you experienced in your life outside of the gym?
- How have others' opinions about you changed?

- Is your spirit a little stronger and have you seen some changes on how you view things or how you feel about life / you / others?
- Are you learning to embrace change and to respect your individual path and journey?
- Does your life look different than it did 8 weeks ago?

KEEP THE MOMENTUM

I loved presenting my 8-Week BLISS™ Body Makeover Program to you, and I've enjoyed sharing my life and my experiences with you. I want you to keep living the BLISS™ lifestyle by building your physical, nutritional and spiritual life.

1. CONTINUE TO TRAIN ON YOUR OWN: Some of you will do very well on your own, I have no doubt! Create your own programs as you go. It's a simple approach but in my view, not usually very successful, especially if you want to continue to improve in your fitness levels and this approach negates the lifestyle aspect of health and wellness – the mental and emotional teachings.

2. HIRE A PERSONAL TRAINER: a better choice. They know what they're doing (most of them, anyway) and they can continue to up the ante as you move through the program with an integrated approach to training and nutrition. Do they have a mental / spiritual lean? Maybe not, but at this point, that may be secondary.

3. JOIN MY HEALTHY LIVING PROGRAM: A truly remarkable, unique and successful monthly program that teaches all of the BLISS™ principals in more depth with workouts, videos, semi-

nars, recipes, diet plans, on-line support and more. For more information, go to www.mccoyfitness.ca and click on **Healthy Living Program**!

4. I also run my popular **10-Week** and **12-Week Best Shape of Your Life Challenge** in which we do up the ante a little bit more for you. I have women all over the world joining… loads of fun! Check them out at www.mccoyfitness.ca

Please make a commitment to yourself to stay healthy and well on all levels. Love and appreciate your body and learn to listen to its inner whisperings and wisdom. Embrace your life, and enjoy your journey. Thanks for journeying with me.

With much love and gratitude,

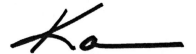

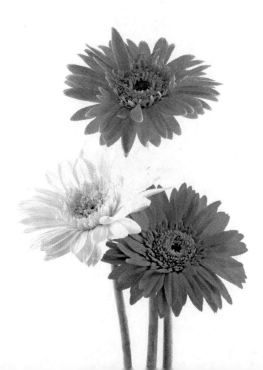

CPSIA information can be obtained at www.ICGtesting.com
Printed in the USA
LVOW071733240512

283171LV00014BA/7/P